A CONCISE GUIDE IN COLOUR

Herbs

by Dr František Stárý
and Dr Václav Jirásek

Illustrated by
František Severa

English Consultant
F. J. Evans, B.Pharm., Ph.D.

Hamlyn
London · New York · Sydney · Toronto

Translated by Olga Kuthanová
Designed and produced by Artia for
The Hamlyn Publishing Group Limited
London – New York – Sydney – Toronto
Astronaut House, Feltham, Middlesex, England

Copyright © 1973 Artia, Prague
Reprinted 1975

ISBN 0 600 31681 5

Printed in Czechoslovakia

CONTENTS

FOREWORD

Man has sought out plants with medicinal properties since time immemorial. Evidence of this are the thousand-year-old traditions and records of popular healing. Even in this age of great development and progress in the fields of chemistry, pharmaceutics and medicine drug plants have lost none of their importance. Over the years scientific research has expanded and made more precise our knowledge of the chemical effect and composition of the active constituents which determine the medicinal properties of plants. It is thus possible to know more about their action and be more exact in prescribing their use in the treatment of various diseases.

The modern pharmaceutical industry makes use of medicinal plants, especially in the dried form as crude drugs and as raw material in the manufacture of medicinal preparations; until such time as the pharmaceutical industry is able to produce the various active substances more economically on a commercial scale, botanical drugs will remain as important as ever. Nevertheless, there is still a large number of medicinal plants in which all the active constituents have not yet been investigated even though their medicinal effect is established by folklore and tradition.

Medicinal plants and the active principles isolated from them are, and will continue to be, an important aid to physicians in their fight against disease. The future development of phytochemistry and medicine is sure to rediscover many a 'forgotten' or hitherto unused plant.

Modern medicine is confronted with an increasing number of diseases connected with the advance of civilization, such as disorder of the circulatory system, infarctions, cancer and infectious diseases caused by all kinds of viruses; medicinal plants — or the active constituents isolated from them — are proving to have marked and, in some cases at least, promising and hopeful effects in the treatment of these diseases.

In this book the reader will find information on medicinal plants presented in terms comprehensible to the layman, including the most important results of scientific research on various individual plants. The general section deals with the significance of medicinal plants, the most important groups of active principles or constituents, the influences which affect their proportion and quality, the forms in which they are used and their methods of application, as well as how to collect, cultivate, harvest, dry and store them.

The pictorial section comprises colour plates of eighty-eight different drug plants with accompanying text. Although there are no detailed botanical descriptions the text includes basic information on the origin and geographic distribution of each plant; besides telling which part of the plant is used for the extraction of the active constituents, how and when it is collected, prepared, dried and stored, an indication is given of the taste and smell. In addition the main active constituents found in the plant are listed, and their effect and use described. Particular attention is given to their current use in medical practice, in some instances also in home remedies, and last of all the text gives information on the use of the plant or its components in the food, cosmetics and other industries. Information on the collection, cultivation and chief commercial sources is also included.

THE IMPORTANCE
OF MEDICINAL PLANTS TODAY

Medicinal plants are a numerically large group of economically important plants. They include various species or cultivated varieties — cultivars — the active constituents of which are used in the treatment of various diseases. This group also includes plants which not only serve a medicinal purpose but contain aromatic substances used in the cosmetics and food industries. Some species of medicinal plants have a primary use outside medicine, being cultivated for the provision of wood, tannins (used in processing leather), plant fibres for the textile industry, and dyes. This latter group, however, is of little importance today as natural dyes have largely been replaced by man-made substances. Other species provide caoutchouc, oil or fodder for domestic animals, or are used by man as vegetables, fruits or ornamental plants. Medicinal plants thus include single-purpose species, used only for their medicinal properties and nothing else, and species that can be put to a number of uses. These are in the majority, their chief application being in fields other than medicine and their use in pharmaceutics secondary or even incidental. Below are some examples.

Species used purely for medicinal purpose include both poisonous and non-poisonous plants. The first group includes such species as Henbane *(Hyoscyamus niger)* and Jimson Weed *(Datura stramonium)*, which contain a group of drugs useful in the treatment of gastric ulcers, as powerful muscle relaxants prior to surgical operations, to control the characteristic tremors of Parkinson's disease and also to prevent travel sickness; European White Hellebore *(Veratrum album)*, used in the treatment of high blood pressure; *Digitalis lanata*, a patent heart poison used in minute doses as a heart tonic; and Ergot Fungus *(Claviceps purpurea)*, which contains a group of chemicals useful in

7

the treatment of migraine. Non-poisonous species include such plants as Restharrow *(Ononis spinosa)*, Ribwort *(Plantago lanceolata)*, Lungwort *(Pulmonaria officinalis)*, Bearberry *(Arctostaphylos uva-ursi)*, and Agrimony *(Agrimonia eupatoria)*. Plants with more widespread uses, although chiefly employed for their herbal properties, include Elder *(Sambucus nigra)*, used also in making refreshing non-alcoholic beverages and home-brewed wines, Blessed Thistle *(Cnicus benedictus)*, used to make liqueurs, Chamomile *(Matricaria chamomilla)*, which is also a source of an essential oil used in the cosmetics industry for bath preparations, and Adonis *(Adonis vernalis)*, a popular rock garden plant which also contains a group of drugs with a very potent action on the failing heart. Then there are the drug plants which have a limited use in medical practice but widespread application in other fields. Examples of these are the Onion *(Allium cepa)*, Garlic *(Allium sativum)*, Chive *(Allium schoenoprasum)*, Horseradish *(Armoracia rusticana)*, Pepper *(Capsicum annuum)*, Parsnip *(Pastinaca sativa)*, and Parsley *(Petroselinum crispum)*, all known for their use in the kitchen, as are Anise *(Anisum vulgare)*, Caraway *(Carum carvi)*, Dill *(Anethum graveolens)*, Coriander *(Coriandrum sativum)*, Garden Thyme *(Thymus vulgaris)* and many others, used mainly as kitchen herbs. Medicinal properties are similarly present in certain purely agricultural plants such as the Opium Poppy *(Papaver somniferum)*, Flax *(Linum usitatissimum)*, Hops *(Humulus lupulus)* and Black Mustard *(Brassica nigra)* which, although used primarily for other purposes, are no less important in the treatment of disease.

One example will suffice as an illustration. The Opium Poppy *(Papaver somniferum)* is a plant cultivated chiefly for its seeds. These are used either for the production of seed oil or else, prepared in various forms, as a cattle feed. Only a small percentage of cultivated poppies is used for the extraction of opium alkaloids, but these are of far greater importance to man — besides being more profitable economically — since they provide modern medicine with its most powerful analgesics, sedatives and antispasmodics.

Even as recently as the first half of the nineteenth century apothecaries not only stocked dried medicinal plants in the form of crude drugs for the preparation of various herbal tea mixtures, but also used them to make all kinds of tinctures, extracts and juices which in turn were employed in preparing medicinal drops, syrups, infusions, ointments and liniments. This period marked not only the peak of the ancient repute of medicinal plants but also the beginning of its decline. This esteem was not unfounded; from the earliest times no other more effective medicinal preparations were available to physicians and drug plants were considered the basis of all treatment. There exist numerous written records and well-authenticated accounts of the collection and cultivation of medicinal plants dating from the beginning of the Christian era and, to a limited extent, from even earlier times. In the Middle Ages knowledge of medicinal plants spread from the monastery garden to the ordinary citizen. Leaving aside the various superstitions and beliefs in supernatural power, popular folk remedies are found in use for the treatment of various illnesses as early as mediaeval times, and even today in many highly developed countries use is still made of numerous different plants, chiefly in the form of teas.

The second half of the nineteenth century brought with it several important discoveries in the newly developing field of chemistry and saw the rapid progress of this science. Medicinal plants became one of its chief objects of interest and in time chemists succeeded in isolating the pure, active substances, or rather groups of substances which they contained and which, in many instances, have replaced the crude drugs. Then came the first synthetic medicines; they became predominant and gradually pushed the herbal medicines which had formerly been used into the background. This trend still continues, even though the once reigning belief that medicinal plants are of no importance and can all be replaced by man-made drugs is no longer tenable. In the same way that drug plants were rapidly falling into disuse a century ago so today they are regaining

9

their rightful place in the field of medicine, though naturally on a far higher level and with a far better knowledge of their effects on the human organism. Researchers are investigating not only the classical plants but also related species that may contain similar active constituents, as well as hitherto unknown plants which have no previous history of medical use.

What importance, then, do medicinal plants have today?

Medicinal plants, or rather the parts that are collected and dried — the crude drugs, for example the roots *(radix)*, leaves *(folium)*, flowers *(flos)*, herbage *(herba)* — are the raw material used for the industrial preparation of pure active substances. The synthetic preparation of many of these substances is either unknown at the present time or uneconomical for industrial purposes. These substances are employed either in their pure form or are used for the preparation of new substances, often with a more significant therapeutic action. Examples of active constituents from plants which are now isolated and used by the medical profession in pure tableted form include quinine from *Cinchona*, the anti-malarial drug, digoxin from *Digitalis lanata* used for the treatment of heart failure and Vinblastine from *Vinca* species used for certain malignant diseases. The organic chemicals from crude drugs also provide a model which can be copied or modified by the organic chemist to produce a more potent drug or a better drug with less side effects. An example of this latter group are the drugs used as local anaesthetics which are based on the artificially modified chemical structure of cocaine. This is a drug isolated from the leaves of a Peruvian bush. Other examples can be found in the penicillin drugs, many of which are semisynthetic but all based on the molecular configuration first isolated from the *Penicillium* fungus.

The following species are examples of important medicinal plants. The drugs used in the treatment of heart disease, for instance, are the cardiac glycosides, natural plant products obtained chiefly from *Digitalis lanata*, Foxglove *(Digitalis purpurea)*, Adonis *(Adonis vernalis)* and Lily-of-the-Valley *(Convallaria majalis)*. Ergot alkaloids obtained from Ergot Fungus

(Claviceps purpurea), either singly or combined, are the basic drugs of obstetrics, internal medicine and neurology. Opium alkaloids, primarily morphine, obtained from the Opium Poppy *(Papaver somniferum)* are contained in the countless pharmaceutical preparations serving to relieve pain, alleviate cramps and suppress bouts of coughing. As yet modern medicine has no substitutes for these natural drugs and physicians cannot do without them.

Medicinal plants, or rather the crude drugs, are used in many instances for the preparation of extracts with water, alcohol or ether — thick, thin, fluid or solid may be produced according to the consistency. Alcoholic extracts are termed tinctures. On occasion these are still obtained from the fresh plant by pressing and subsequent thickening of the juice *(succus)*. All these 'galenicals' — medicinal preparations made by extracting the desired constituent from the crude drug according to the Galenic method, a technique introduced by Claudius Galen, a Greek physician of the second century AD — are of minor importance today. However, there are still a number of drugs from which the various pure active principles have not been isolated or where the combination of their active elements has a much more powerful therapeutic action. For instance, an excellent preparation in the treatment of nervous disorders is the tincture or extract made from Valerian *(Valeriana officinalis)*. The alcoholic extract from a mixture of the leaves of Bogbean *(Menyanthes trifoliata)*, the top parts of Centaury *(Centaurium minus)*, the seed vessels of Bitter Orange *(Citrus aurantium)*, and the roots of Gentian *(Gentiana lutea)* plus a small quantity of cinnamon oil yields the well-known bitter tincture 'Tinctura amara', an excellent and classic medicine in the treatment of digestive disorders. Similarly, various extracts are used in the preparation of capsules. Compared with commercially produced, ready-made tablets and pills, capsules have the advantage of being made up individually according to a physician's or herbalist's prescription and of containing the various constituents in the proportion he considers most beneficial for a particular patient.

11

Drugs from medicinal plants are the basic material for making up herbal tea mixtures, taken either in the form of a decoction or as an infusion. Medicinal teas are of varied composition according to which disease they are intended to treat. They serve as an auxiliary medicine, that is, their mild physiological action promotes that of the primary medicinal preparation. In some instances, especially in chronic ailments, their action is even more effective than that of fast-acting medicines.

Typical drug plants used in herbal tea mixtures are Elderberry *(Sambucus nigra)*, Birch *(Betula verrucosa)*, Blessed Thistle *(Cnicus benedictus)*, Mullein *(Verbascum thapsiforme)*, Chamomile *(Matricaria chamomilla)*, Hawthorn *(Crataegus oxyacantha)* Common Juniper *(Juniperus communis)*, Restharrow *(Ononis spinosa)*, Ribwort *(Plantago lanceolata)*, Small-leaved Lime *(Tilia cordata)*, Peppermint *(Mentha × piperita)*, Bearberry *(Arctostaphylos uva-ursi)*, various species of *Artemisia*, Marsh Mallow *(Althaea officinalis)*, Garden Sage *(Salvia officinalis)*, *Herniaria glabra*, *Drosera rotundifolia*, Agrimony *(Agrimonia eupatoria)*, St John's Wort *(Hypericum perforatum)* and Centaury *(Centaurium minus)*.

Medicinal plants are also becoming an important addition to certain industrial food products, especially dietetic preparations; the plants chiefly used are those which contain aromatic substances, vitamins, and important amino acids and enzymes to aid digestion and promote certain body functions.

The plant kingdom is a limitless source of new species of plants containing active constituents of therapeutic value, and scientists throughout the world are well aware of this. That is why scientific expeditions are organized and extensive tests made on the pharmacological activities of the little-known plants so collected. An example of the results of such efforts is the discovery of reserpine, an alkaloid which has a hypotensive effect, that is, it lowers blood pressure. This was discovered in plants of the genus *Rauwolfia*. Hypotensive alkaloids have also been discovered in the European evergreen Periwinkle *(Vinca minor)* of the genus *Catharanthus*, together with an alkaloid which is useful in the treatment of certain types of malignant disease.

Moreover, new specific active constituents have been discovered even in well known and much used drug plants, for instance, chamomile oil (the oil of *Matricaria chamomilla*) was found to contain principles with specific anti-inflammatory effects (chamazulene and bisabolol). Members of the Carrot family, (Umbelliferae), have yielded numerous substances of the furocoumarin group that hold promise for use in internal medicine.

Medicinal plants and the investigation of their chemical composition as well as their therapeutic effects yield knowledge used in the synthetic preparation of new substances or provide substances which in various combinations become powerful medicinal agents.

Thus, for instance, from ergotamine, an alkaloid of Ergot Fungus *(Claviceps purpurea)*, it is possible to obtain by chemical means the semi-synthetic alkaloid dihydroergotamine which is very effective in the treatment of migraine. Certain members of the Nightshade family (Solanaceae) and of the family Dioscoreaceae contain glyco-alkaloids — solasodine, tomatidine, diosgenine, for example — which serve for the synthetic preparation of steroid hormones, previously isolated only from animal organs or products.

Lastly, drug plants are of economic importance and a profitable commercial product. As long as they were gathered wild the amount collected could only be small, although the price they commanded was much higher than that paid for other plant products. All this was changed, however, with the introduction of large-scale crop production of industrially important species which produced equally large economic profits. In some countries, therefore, drug plants have become a significant market commodity.

Little more needs to be said about the present-day importance of medicinal plants for it will be apparent from the foregoing that the plants themselves, either in the form of crude drugs or, even more important, for the medically active materials isolated from them, have been, are and always will be an important aid to the physician in the treatment of disease.

THE MAIN GROUPS OF ACTIVE PRINCIPLES OR CONSTITUENTS OBTAINED FROM MEDICINAL PLANTS

The therapeutic agents in medicinal plants are certain specific groups of substances or individual substances which are the products of plant metabolism. Active principles may be divided into two main groups: toxic — those that have a poisonous effect on animal organisms — and non-toxic — those that do not cause poisoning but are therapeutically effective. Needless to say, it is impossible to draw a precise dividing line between the two, for even certain non-toxic plants — aromatic species containing essential oil, for example — may, if used in excessive quantities or over a longer period than that prescribed, impair the function of various bodily organs. The symptoms of mild poisoning, such as sickness, diarrhoea or pains in the stomach or intestines, are not fatal but may be unpleasant or painful. Only those plants that are clearly poisonous when taken even in minute quantities can be definitely branded as toxic; in the pictorial section of this book attention is drawn to the fact that they are poisonous and should not be gathered except by a qualified collector who knows how to take the necessary precautions when gathering them. It is dangerous for any patient to attempt to treat himself with such a drug without the advice and attendant care of a physician. Acutely poisonous plants are used in the treatment of disease in very small doses. They are extremely dangerous in non-qualified hands because the dosage required to achieve the beneficial effect is very close to the dosage which produces symptoms of poisoning. On the other hand, when used by experienced doctors even extremely toxic substances can serve to restore man's health.

The principal groups of active constituents are described below. Besides these the plants also contain subsidiary components which sometimes serve to increase the efficiency of their therapeutically important principles. An example of this action, which is known as synergism, is to be found in laxative drugs, which contain anthraquinone glycosides, such as Senna *(Cassia acutifolia)* or Cascara *(Rhamnus purshiana)*.

ALKALOIDS

Alkaloids are naturally occurring materials in some plant tissues and are distinguished chemically by the fact that they contain nitrogen. They have marked toxic effects on animal organisms. In the main they are stable, crystalline substances that are both odourless and colourless and also sensitive to high temperatures, at which they disintegrate. Rarely does a plant contain one alkaloid only; generally it contains a group of chemically related components. The responses produced by alkaloids in animals and plants have been studied in some detail and it has been found that alkaloids rank among the most efficient and therapeutically most significant substances known. They generally occur in all the plant organs but their concentration varies and appears to be greatest just before or at the beginning of the flowering period. So far no satisfactory answer has been found to the question of their function in the life cycle of the plant. It has been suggested by some scientists that they are waste substances, while others consider them to have hormonal activity or possibly even metabolic function, participating in the biochemical reactions of plant cells.

Several hundred alkaloids are known to modern science. The first alkaloid was isolated in 1803 by Friedrich Wilhelm Adam Sertürner (1793—1841), a pharmacist's assistant in the German town of Paderborn. It was morphine, the basic alkaloid from opium. This was followed by the isolation of further plant alkaloids, such as strychnine (1818), quinine (1820), coniine (1827), nicotine (1828), atropine, hyoscyamine and colchicine (1833).

Many of the plant species presented in this book are significant because of their alkaloid content. They are plants that are either indigenous to the Old World or became established there after being introduced from overseas centuries ago, such plants as Jimson Weed *(Datura stramonium)* and Pepper *(Capsicum annuum)*, for example. Henbane *(Hyoscyamus niger)*, and Deadly Nightshade *(Atropa belladonna)* are typical alkaloidal plants which contain a group of alkaloids chemically related to the substance tropane. Examples are atropine, hyoscyamine and scopolamine, constituents which significantly affect smooth muscle and thereby bring about the relaxation of muscular spasms. They are also of importance in internal medicine and ophthalmology. Smooth muscle is sometimes known as involuntary muscle because voluntary control of its contractions is not possible. Smooth muscle is found in internal organs of the body such as the bladder and womb. Another typical alkaloidal plant is the Opium Poppy *(Papaver somniferum)*, which besides morphine, narcotine, papaverine, codeine and thebaine contains some twenty more alkaloids of lesser medicinal importance. Alkaloids from Opium Poppy are very effective in relieving pain, relaxing cramps and diminishing or suppressing the desire to cough. Ergot Fungus *(Claviceps purpurea)* is another important alkaloidal plant. Ergot alkaloids are widely used by gynaecologists, neurologists and psychiatrists. Mention should also be made of the European White Hellebore *(Veratrum album)*, Autumn Crocus *(Colchicum autumnale)*, Monkshood *(Aconitum napellus)* and Greater Celandine *(Chelidonium majus)*. Toxic alkaloids such as morphine, codeine or colchicine are taken in the purified form as tablets or as ingredients of liquid preparations such as mixtures and tinctures. Other alkaloids such as ergotamine and atropine may also be injected for rapid onset of action.

GLYCOSIDES

Glycosides occur naturally in plants and are characterized by the fact that chemically they consist of a sugar portion attached by a special chemical bond to a non-sugar portion. They are readily broken down by the mediation of enzymes into these two parts. Glycosides are substances with a pronounced physiological action on animal tissues and are poisonous to man. They are the product of special metabolic processes in certain plants. Their concentration in the various plant organs varies and is dependent on the age, or ecology, of the plant. Those with the most significant therapeutic action are the cardiac glycosides. They exert effects on the muscle tissue of the heart, which consists of specially modified hard-working muscle cells.

During the disease known as congestive heart failure, or dropsy, the heart muscle becomes inefficient and the heart enlarged. The cardiac glycosides increase the efficiency of the failing heart and return its size to normal. They are often referred to as digitalis glycosides after the plants of the genus *Digitalis* of which they are characteristic constituents.

Cardiac glycosides are present, for example, in *Digitalis lanata*, the Foxglove *(Digitalis purpurea)*, and other species of this genus, and also in such plants as Adonis *(Adonis vernalis)* and Lily-of-the-Valley *(Convallaria majalis)*. Although already long known to the Irish as a popular home remedy the uses of *Digitalis* in cardiology were not acknowledged by the medical profession until 1785 when the Birmingham physician William Withering published his report on its uses in diseases associated with the heart. The plant he first used was the Foxglove *(Digitalis purpurea)*, which is indigenous to England and western Europe: in the 1930s, however, its use was replaced almost entirely on the continent by *Digitalis lanata* from the Balkans. Cardiac glycosides are natural plant products that are irreplaceable in current medical therapy. They are very potent even in small doses and extremely poisonous. The most commonly used drug in this group is digoxin from *Digitalis lanata* which is commonly prescribed in the form of small tablets. The main problem associated with the use of *Digitalis* is the fact that the useful or beneficial dose is close to the toxic dose. Symptoms of toxicity will be observed by the physician as side effects. This arises because the glycosides are only slowly eliminated from the body; for this reason the lanatosides are sometimes used because they are more easily excreted.

Another important group of glycosides from the medical viewpoint are the anthraquinone glycosides which occur in a fairly small number of plant families, for example, Rhamnaceae, Polygonaceae and Rubiaceae. They are mildly poisonous in larger doses and are generally used for their laxative action in certain disorders of the digestive system. The anthraquinone glycosides have been much abused by the general public as daily laxatives. This regular use of laxatives has been shown to be harmful to the natural rhythm of the body and leads to laziness of the bowels. There are instances, however, when it is necessary to use a laxative, for example, before surgery, during pregnancy or before X-ray of the intestine, and in these cases the anthraquinone glycosides, owing to their mild action, are preferred. Of the plants dealt with in the pictorial section of this book anthraquinone glycosides are present in Rhubarb *(Rheum palmatum)* and Madder Root *(Rubia tinctorum)*.

A therapeutic action is also exerted by the 'mustard' or thiocyanate glycosides. They are very unstable, being readily broken down by the mediation of an appropriate enzyme which is also present in the plant. Mustard glycosides are distinguished chemically by the presence of sulphur in their structure. They occur chiefly in the families Cruciferae, Tropaeolaceae and Resedaceae, and exert an irritant and disinfectant action besides improving the blood supply to various organs. Applied externally in large doses they cause marked local irritation and even inflammation of the skin. Two examples of such glycosides are sinigrin, found in Black Mustard *(Brassica nigra)*, and glucotropaeolin, present in *Tropaeolum majus*.

Then there are the phenolic glycosides which are only slightly poisonous and exert a disinfectant, anti-inflammatory and diuretic action. They are present in many species of the family Ericaceae. Of the plants depicted in this book, two in which these glycosides occur are Bearberry *(Arctostaphylos uva-ursi)*, which contains arbutin and methylarbutin, and Cowslip *(Primula veris)*, of the family Primulaceae, which contains primulaverin and primaverin.

SAPONINS

Saponins are natural compounds which have a chemical nature very similar to that of the glycosides but are distinguished by the fact that they produce a soapy lather when shaken with water. Their most marked physiological activity is that they cause the break up of red blood cells, and are therefore potent blood poisons. This process is known as haemolysis. Saponins have a marked irritant effect and some are extremely toxic, such as those occurring in *Paris quadrifolia* and *Agrostemma githago*. However, they also have beneficial therapeutic properties and may act as an expectorant in catarrh of the upper respiratory passages. They are often found together with glycosides. *Digitalis lanata*, for example, in addition to cardiac glycosides also contains the saponin tigonin, and Foxglove *(Digitalis purpurea)* the saponins digitonin and gitonin.

Saponins are present in most species of *Primula* and also in many members of the family Solanaceae. The Horse Chestnut *(Aesculus hippocastanum)*, contains the saponin aescin.

ESSENTIAL OILS

Essential oils are liquid components of plant cells that are volatile and as a rule have a pleasant fragrance. Chemically their principal constituents are a group of complex substances known as terpenes and their compounds or derivatives. They generally occur in special cells or glands where they accumulate possibly as waste products. This is a typical characteristic of many of the families noted for their content of essential oils, for example Pinaceae, Labiatae, Myrtaceae, Rutaceae and Umbelliferae.

Essential oils are substances with multiple effects. They exert an antiseptic action in that they check the growth of germs. Well known, for instance, are the marked germicidal properties of thymol, a constituent of the essential oils of Garden Thyme *(Thymus vulgaris)* and Wild Thyme *(T. serpyllum)*. These are extensively used in mouth washes and gargles. Antiseptic properties are also exhibited by the essential oil of Garlic *(Allium sativum)* and Onion *(Allium cepa)*. These are well established remedies for bronchitis and the common cold. The action of essential oils in the treatment of mycoses, scabies and other skin diseases caused by parasites, is also well known. Anethol, a constituent of the oil of Anise *(Anisum vulgare)*, has a marked odour that repels certain insects. The anthelminthic action of certain volatile oils is also well established. A more detailed account of the effects of the various essential oils will be found in the descriptions accompanying the plates in the pictorial section of this book.

Some essential oils irritate the skin, and in many cases cause inflammation and even swelling. Administered in therapeutic doses, however, they cause a marked increase in the blood supply and many are, therefore, used as a constituent of anti-rheumatic liniments. The oil of Black Mustard *(Brassica nigra)*, for instance, is used in this way. Also significant are the properties of reducing inflammation and counteracting fever of certain volatile oils contained, for example, in Chamomile *(Matricaria chamo-*

milla), Milfoil *(Achillea millefolium)* and Peppermint *(Mentha ×
piperita)*.

Individual constituents of essential oils, such as eugenol,
camphor and menthol, have an anaesthetic effect. Others, like
camphor and borneol, affect heart muscle and the circulatory
system, producing a stimulation. Essential oils also affect the
central nervous system and are used as stimulants, sedatives
and even narcotics. Plants containing these types of essential
oils include Valerian *(Valeriana officinalis)* and Common Balm
(Melissa officinalis).

The smooth muscles are influenced by a number of essential
oils. Most of these exert a favourable action on the digestive
system — both the liver and gall bladder as well as the stomach
and intestines. The effects of oil of Peppermint *(Mentha × piperita)*, Anise *(Anisum vulgare)*, and Caraway *(Carum carvi)* are well
known. Their constituents stimulate the flow of gastric secretions, alleviate digestive disorders, stimulate the appetite, and
the secretion of bile.

Some essential oils have an undesirable effect on the womb
in that they increase the blood supply to this organ and may
cause miscarriage in pregnancy. Particularly dangerous are
certain constituents of essential oils such as apiol and myristicine.
On the other hand many of these components have excellent
diuretic properties and also exert an antiseptic action in the
urinary passages, such as the oil of Restharrow *(Ononis spinosa)*
and Parsley *(Petroselinum crispum)*, for example.

Other oils have a favourable effect on the upper respiratory
passages and have a wide medicinal use in this connection, for
example, the oils of Garden and Wild Thyme *(Thymus vulgaris
and T. serpyllum)*.

Many of the essential oils are important components of
flavouring which enhance the taste and aroma of food and
ncrease the enjoyment of a meal. Their favourable effect on
the digestive processes is an additional benefit. Fresh herbs,
or rather their roots, leaves, flowers and fruits, are sometimes
used but generally they are employed in dried form, whole or

crushed. For culinary purposes, however, fresh herbs always have a better aroma. If dried material is used it should be freshly ground to a powder to conserve as many of the volatile principles as possible. When possible herbs should be added to a dish towards the end of the cooking time and the vessel should have a tight-fitting lid to help retain the flavour and aroma.

The food industry — the producers of beverages, both alcoholic and non-alcoholic, are included in this grouping — also use volatile oils extensively as flavouring and perfuming agents, and they are employed in the same way by the confectionery and tobacco trades. Today essential oils are generally isolated from the fresh or dried plants on an industrial scale.

BITTER PRINCIPLES

Bitter principles are non-poisonous, non-nitrogenous substances of varied chemical composition but with one characteristic in common — their strong bitter, but not unpleasant, taste. They occur in various plant families, such as Gentianaceae, Compositae and Labiatae.

They are generally used in medicine in the form of alcoholic extracts, tinctures and medicinal wines. Taken before meals as prescribed they stimulate the appetite by promoting the flow of digestive secretions and thereby aid the digestion itself. They are also administered to convalescents for their sedative and tonic properties.

Of the plants presented in the pictorial section of this book those that contain bitter principles are chiefly Blessed Thistle *(Cnicus benedictus)*, Yellow Gentian *(Gentiana lutea)* and other *Gentiana* species, Bogbean *(Menyanthes trifoliata)* and Centaury *(Centaurium minus)*. All species of *Artemisia* are also rich in bitter principles. The bitter drugs are an important ingredient in the production of various aperitifs such as vermouths and of stomach bitters. The most famous bitter, hops, is used in the production of English beer and ale.

TANNINS

Tannins are organic, non-nitrogenous plant products which have astringent properties. They are soluble in water and alcohol. Exposed to air they turn dark, their composition changes and they lose their effective properties. It will therefore be obvious that tannin drugs lose their beneficial properties if stored for long periods. Plant families rich in tannins include Rosaceae, Geraniaceae and Papilionaceae. Members of the families Cruciferae and Papaveraceae, on the other hand, are totally devoid of tannins.

Tannins are of medical significance because of their astringent properties; these promote rapid healing and the formation of new tissue on wounds and inflamed mucosa. They are used in the treatment of varicose ulcers, haemorrhoids, minor burns and frostbite as well as inflammation of the gums. Internally they are administered in cases of diarrhoea and intestinal catarrh. Tannins occur in crude drugs either as the chief active principle, for example, in the bark of Oak *(Cortex quercus)* or the leaves of Bilberry *(Folium myrtilli)*, or as subsidiary components which increase the effectiveness of the main active principles as in Peppermint *(Mentha × piperita)* and Garden Sage *(Salvia officinalis)*. On the other hand, their presence in Bearberry *(Arctostaphylos uva-ursi)* is a disadvantage.

Tannins are also widely used in industry for the conversion of hides into leather.

MUCILAGES

Mucilages are products of metabolic activity in plants. They consist of chains of chemically linked sugars known as polysaccharides, partially soluble in water in which they will swell and form a gel. It is for this reason that drugs which exhibit this property are called mucilaginous. Mucilages are employed medicinally for their local action, that is their beneficial effect on diseased tissue at the point of contact. For example, mucilaginous drugs exert a favourable action in catarrh of the upper respiratory passages in that they soothe abraded mucous membrane and diminish irritation. Their effect in the intestines is also excellent. Not only do they check undesirable or fermentation processes but they also promote a mild laxative action due to the initiation of regular, rhythmic peristalsis. These properties are employed in pediatrics, for example, in the treatment of intestinal disorders in infants.

Some of the more important mucilaginous drugs presented in the pictorial section of this book include the roots and leaves of Marsh Mallow *(Radix et Folium althaeae)*, the flowers of Common Mallow *(Flos malvae)*, Flax seed *(Semen lini)*, Iceland Moss *(Cetraria islandica)*, and Plantain seed *(Semen psyllium)* of the species *Plantago psyllium* and *Plantago indica*. In some medicinal plants, such as Mullein *(Verbascum thapsiforme)*, mucilages are not the chief active constituent but are of therapeutic importance as auxiliary components promoting the action of the main active principle.

Medicines from mucilaginous drugs are prepared by extraction in cold water for boiling causes them to lose their efficacy.

OTHER GROUPS OF ACTIVE PRINCIPLES

Besides the main groups already described, there are several other groups of active principles which are just as important both chemically and therapeutically. These include the following:

Organic acids, which play an important role in the medicinal properties of many plants. The chief ones are malic acid, citric acid, oxalic acid and tartaric acid. They have a mild laxative effect.

Sugars, which are important auxiliary substances in many plants. The large group of substances to which the sugars belong also includes the mucilages previously mentioned and other polysaccharides, such as starch.

Mention should also be made of *plant oils* and *vitamins*. The plant oils are useful dietary components in place of animal fats as it is thought by some experts that they have a beneficial effect in the prevention of heart disease and diseases of the body arteries. Vitamins, which are abundant in plant tissues, are essential for the maintenance of health.

Plants, however, have not as yet been fully used in medicine, nor have their pharmacological properties been thoroughly investigated. Pharmacognosists and pharmacologists have much to work on for the flora of Asia, Africa, South America and Australia is still largely unknown and may perhaps yield new and important discoveries that will prove to be of great medicinal value.

SHOULD DRUG PLANTS
BE CULTIVATED OR COLLECTED WILD?

The title of this chapter raises a question which is still an object of controversy, since there are two distinct opinions on the matter. Adherents of one view believe that drug plants collected wild in their natural habitat are more effective than those cultivated commercially as crops, whereas opponents of this belief support the contrary opinion. Neither the one nor the other is totally correct, for as the situation stands at present those plants that man has not been able to cultivate with success, such as Monkshood *(Aconitum napellus)*, European White Hellebore *(Veratrum album)*, Autumn Crocus *(Colchicum autumnale)*, and *Herniaria glabra*, are collected wild, as are those species where single-purpose cultivation would be uneconomic, for example Elderberry *(Sambucus nigra)*, Common Oak *(Quercus robur)*, Small-leaved Lime *(Tilia cordata)* and Common Juniper *(Juniperus communis)*, and last of all those species which require such a specialized environment for growth as is impossible to provide in normal cultivation, such as Sundew *(Drosera rotundifolia)*, Bogbean *(Menyanthes trifoliata)*, Iceland Moss *(Cetraria islandica)*, and Mistletoe *(Viscum album)*.

Plants that are grown commercially include those that have been under cultivation for centuries, for example Anise *(Anisum vulgare)*, Onion *(Allium cepa)*, Fennel *(Foeniculum vulgare)*, Caraway *(Carum carvi)*, Pepper *(Capsicum annuum)*, and Opium Poppy *(Papaver somniferum)*, as well as those that are in such demand as crude drugs that their collection in the wild is not sufficient to satisfy the requirements of the pharmaceutical industry, among them medicinal plants which are basic pharmaceutical materials such as Chamomile *(Matricaria chamomilla)*, *Digitalis lanata*, Ergot Fungus *(Claviceps purpurea)*, Valerian *(Valeriana officinalis)*, and Marsh Mallow *(Althaea officinalis)*.

Also cultivated are rare species with a limited distribution in the wild, such as Adonis *(Adonis vernalis)* and Gentian *(Gentiana lutea)*, and those with a distribution so sparse and scattered as to preclude the collection of sufficient quantities: Blessed Thistle *(Cnicus benedictus)* and Elecampane *(Inula helenium)*, for example. Lastly, there are, of course, those plants that are comparatively easy to cultivate and where commercial cultivation promises to be profitable, as in the case of Ribwort *(Plantago lanceolata)*, Common Balm *(Melissa officinalis)*, and Madder Root *(Rubia tinctorum)*, for instance.

Apart from plants which are purely cultivated crops, all other medicinal plants are obtained both by collection in the wild and from cultivation.

Until recently it was thought that there was no difference between the concentration of active principles in cultivated plants and those collected wild, provided that the wild herbs were healthy and well developed, free of disease and insect pests and gathered at the appropriate time, and that the crude drugs were properly prepared, dried and stored. Recent research has, however, brought to light the problems of the existence of chemical races in certain species of medicinal plants. Medicinal plants are the subject of careful chemical study by pharmacognosists, and with the advantages of modern breeding and cultivation methods it soon became clear that within a given species plants which had the same external appearance (phenotype) could have chemical compositions which differed considerably. It has also become evident that these differences are inherited, in other words they are genetic differences and not due solely to differences in environment. This has enabled certain strains (genotypes) to be selected which are high yielding in desirable chemical constituents. These are bred and cultivated for medicinal purposes. It is evident that in wild populations from different localities the medicinal properties may vary greatly, thereby creating problems of administration and dosage. Examples of chemical races may be found in *Digitalis* species, Jimson Weed *(Datura stramonium)* and Rhubarb *(Rheum palmatum)*.

Today, apart from those species which cannot be cultivated successfully, collection of medicinal plants in the wild is inefficient and generally unprofitable for the picker. Collection in the wild is mostly carried out in countries with an ample labour force and limited job opportunities, for example, in areas with little industry. In industrially developed countries drug plants are either cultivated or imported.

There is no doubt that cultivation has numerous advantages. Plants grown in a single consolidated area give a high yield, facilitate the control of insects and disease, permit mechanization — and therefore speedy and planned harvesting — as well as mass transport to the drying sheds. Cultivation produces plants of uniform quality, which can be fed, watered and treated as necessary, and an end product — the crude drug — that is pure and unadulterated by admixtures of any kind.

Collection in the wild cannot guarantee these advantages and that is why preference is given to cultivation of drug plants wherever possible. Many of the crude drugs described in this book are poisonous and can be found growing wild. The dangers of collection by the general public are obvious, because even experts have difficulty in the correct identification of some species unless they are in flower. In the dried or powdered form crude drugs can only be identified by an experienced pharmacognosist using a high-powered microscope. The basis of such identifications is the fact that plants have characteristic arrangements of cells and structures when prepared and viewed under the microscope. Mistaken identity during collection, particularly of plants with similar-shaped leaves such as Mullein and Foxglove, could lead to cases of accidental poisoning.

Very few drugs are collected or cultivated in this country, with the exception of some kitchen herbs. They are obtained chiefly from cultivated varieties imported from the USA and Europe. The purchase of herbal remedies from a registered pharmacist or herbalist will ensure that the correct substance of a standard potency is obtained.

PRACTICES AND PROCEDURES
OF DRUG COLLECTION AND PREPARATION

Whether growing wild or under cultivation only certain parts, or rather organs, of the plant are collected as the commercial drug. These are differentiated as follows:

1. the underground parts, namely the root *(radix)*, rhizome *(rhizoma)*, tuber *(tuber)* and bulb *(bulbus)*.

2. everything above ground — the aerial parts — such as the leaf *(folium)*, herbage *(herba)*, flower *(flos)*, fruit *(fructus)*, seed *(semen)*, and bark *(cortex)*.

In the pictorial section of this book the text accompanying each plate tells which part is collected. Only exceptionally is the whole plant harvested. Of the higher plants this is true in the case of Sundew *(Drosera rotundifolia)* and Mistletoe *(Viscum album)*. In this higher category the entire plant is usually not harvested because the active principles are generally more concentrated in a specific organ or organs and collection of the whole plant would simply result in an undesirable 'dilution' of the active principles. A further important factor influencing the quality of the drug is the time at which it is harvested. It is well known that the concentration of active constituents varies during the life cycle of a plant. A young, germinating plant usually contains the lowest amount of the principles used for medicinal purposes. This concentration gradually increases and is usually at its highest during the flowering stage, after which it again declines. This very simplified 'rule', however, has its exceptions and that is why the best time for collecting is also specified for each species.

In the case of lower plants, such as Ergot Fungus and Iceland Moss, which do not have specific organs, the whole plant is harvested.

Various plant products such as balsams, resins, and gums are also gathered. In the main these are substances exuded by a plant when injured. In this book there is only one example of such a drug, namely opium — the dried, milky latex exuded from the capsules of the Opium Poppy *(Papaver somniferum)* when incised.

COLLECTION

The general rules for collecting the various parts of a plant are as follows:

Roots of annual plants are usually not collected. Those of biennials are generally harvested in the autumn of the first year's growth, or in the spring before the beginning of the second year's growth. This is because the roots are storage organs for the plant and accumulate active principles during the summer months. The roots and rhizomes of perennials are gathered in the same period; those of slow-growing plants are harvested in the second or third year of growth or even later. This applies to the majority of drug plants collected in the wild. In the case of cultivated plants the grower cannot afford to leave a field crop in the ground for a number of years as this would prove uneconomic. The roots of Deadly Nightshade *(Atropa belladonna)* and Valerian *(Valeriana officinalis)*, for instance, are therefore harvested at the end of one year only, even though the yield is not as large as when crops are left in the ground for several years. It is not always true that roots of older plants are better for they generally rot and disintegrate, as is the case with cultivated Rhubarb *(Rheum palmatum)*, Gentian *(Gentiana lutea)* and Deadly Nightshade *(Atropa belladonna)*.

Tubers should be harvested during the flowering period because this aids the identification of the species. Typical plants with the active principles concentrated chiefly in the tubers are Monkshood *(Aconitum napellus)* and various species of *Orchis*.

These are not included in this book but are an important drug containing as much as fifty per cent mucilage *(Tubera salep)*.

Bulbs are collected at the end of the flowering period, best of all when the leaves of the plant are just beginning to die off. Examples of this group are the Onion *(Allium cepa)* and Garlic *(Allium sativum)*. An important drug of this type is the Sea Onion *(Urginea maritima)*, which is indigenous in the Mediterranean area. It contains important cardiac glycosides which are used not only for medicinal purposes but also to exterminate rodents, especially brown rats. It is comparatively non-poisonous to household pets, but the bulbs are very bitter and in most animals produce vomiting as part of a protective reflex.

Leaves are gathered throughout the whole growing period, as a rule, for a single harvest usually does not yield a drug of good value. Young leaves are thought to be of the highest quality as the content of active principles in the actively growing parts is highest.

Herbage (the aerial or top parts of the plant) is collected with the flower-bearing stems just before or at the beginning of the flowering stage, for when in full bloom the fruits are already partially developed and their presence is not desirable in the crude drug. In recent years crude drugs from the top parts and flowering heads of plants are replacing those from leaves, wherever the quality is sufficient, because their collection is much easier and therefore more economic. This is usual with Common Balm *(Melissa officinalis)* and Peppermint *(Mentha × piperita)*.

Flowers or the whole *inflorescences* are gathered at the beginning of the flowering period. Full-blown blossoms or ones that are past their prime are not suitable for the drug market because they disintegrate easily and are of unsatisfactory quality.

Fruits and *seeds* are collected when mature. In the case of cultivated crops, which are harvested by machine, this is done just before they are fully ripe so that the fruits do not crumble or the seeds fall out in the field. They are then generally left to ripen in sheaves in the field or in the barn prior to threshing, being transported in canvas sheets to prevent loss.

Bark is collected either in spring, when the trees and shrubs begin to bud, or in autumn after they have shed their leaves. These are the times of the year when the flow of sap is at a maximum and the bark readily detached from the wood.

The method of collection and the time of harvest is different for each of the various parts.

Roots and *rhizomes* are dug up with special implements, often specifically adapted for a particular species, or ploughed up when the plants are cultivated as a crop. Prior to drying the thin, adventitious roots and remainders of the aerial parts, soil and any other extraneous matter are removed by hand. If this cannot be done by shaking, then the roots are placed on a wire mesh and the soil removed with a hose. Whichever method has been used, all the roots are subsequently washed thoroughly and sometimes scrubbed with a brush as well; when the water has dripped off any fleshy roots are cut in half with a knife or into smaller pieces by special cutting machines and then dried. *Rhizomes* and *tubers* are prepared by the same method. *Bulbs* are not washed, but prior to drying the fine roots, wilted or dried top parts, and the dry outer skins are removed. Nowadays the bulbs of cultivated plants are harvested, at least in part, by mechanical means.

Leaves are either picked singly or else the entire stem is cut off and the leaves afterwards stripped. Leaves harvested for the drug market should be full grown, healthy and free from disease and insect pests, and clean and dry, without any trace of moisture from dew or rain.

Aerial parts are cut off several centimetres above the ground; for cultivated crops use is sometimes made of specially adapted harvesting machines. In the case of old mature plants where the bottom section of the stems have already become woody, only the non-woody parts are collected.

Flowers are generally picked by hand. The flower heads only of certain plants of the family Compositae, such as Chamomile *(Matricaria chamomilla)*, are harvested with the aid of special combs, much like those used to gather blueberries or cranberries. Mechanized equipment for this purpose is still in the development stage.

Fruits and *seeds* are picked by hand, for example those of Common Juniper *(Juniperus communis)*, or harvested with the same type of combine harvester used for cereal grains. This method is employed with cultivated crops such as Anise *(Anisum vulgare)*, Fennel *(Foeniculum vulgare)*, Caraway *(Carum carvi)*, Coriander *(Coriandrum sativum)* and Flax *(Linum usitatissimum)*.

Bark is collected by hand. It is stripped from the trunk or branches after it has first been cut and tapped; this is best carried out after rain rather than in very dry weather. Three- to four-year-old branches are best suited for this purpose, rather than one-year growths or thick, old branches where the bark has already cracked.

It is of vital importance in the collection of drug plants that they should be delivered to the drying shed as rapidly as possible, care being taken that they are not packed too tightly and that they do not 'sweat' during transport. Otherwise there is the danger of an undesirable chemical change in the composition of the active principles. After collection enzymes present in the plant cells will start to break down the active principles. Sugars and glycosides are particularly susceptible to this type of deterioration with a consequent loss of potency.

In the case of Foxglove *(Digitalis purpurea)* and Senna *(Cassia acutifolia)*, potent natural glycosides known as primary glycosides are broken down by the removal of a sugar component to artificial products known as secondary glycosides with some loss of potency and therapeutic efficacy. In the case of Cascara *(Rhamnus purshiana)* the opposite is true because the secondary glycosides produced by storage are more effective when used as a laxative than the fresh plant. The crude drug is the end product of the drying process. It is stored whole, cut into parts of a given size, or ground into a powder.

DRYING

Drying is a very important process in that it transforms the parts of the fresh plant collected into the crude drug. If properly dried the drug retains most of its original colour. This is a very simple criterion for judging a dried sample of a herb and thereby the quality of the drug, but it is generally correct. Drying, a process by which water is removed from the plant thus preventing spoilage, is the simplest method of preservation. The fresh drug materials should be dried in airy, dry, and well-ventilated premises, usually on rust-free steel-meshed or firm fabric-meshed frames. It should be unnecessary to point out that these premises must be spotlessly clean, free of dust and protected against mice and the entry of household animals. Larger quantities of drug plants must be dried in industrial drying sheds. The method of drying and type of drying room depends on the plant species and the parts to be dried. Drying should be as rapid as possible and to prevent needless crumbling the raw material should be handled no more than absolutely necessary. When dried on frames the plants should be spread out in thin layers to speed drying and to prevent spoilage by moisture condensation and overheating. In some cases the aerial parts are tied in bunches and hung up to dry. One of the essential requirements for drying is perfect air circulation which must be provided by adequate ventilation. The duration of the drying process is governed by what parts of the plant are being dried — whether they have a high or low moisture content — and the drying temperature. Flowers and leaves dry more quickly than herbage, while roots, rhizomes and tubers take the longest. The drug is properly dried when it breaks easily, in the case of leaves not only the blade but also the central and lateral veins, in the case of top parts both the leaves and stems.

Selection of the correct drying temperature is most important in determining the quality of the drug. Best quality drugs are generally obtained by natural drying in the shade coupled with good air circulation. Artificial drying in special rooms where space is limited requires higher temperatures. These, however, must be such as to preserve the drug's quality by retaining the maximum possible content of active principles, since some components deteriorate or vaporize at high temperatures. Plants containing volatile oils, for instance, must be dried at temperatures not exceeding 40°C because these oils vaporize easily at higher temperatures and their concentration in the drug is markedly diminished. Drug plants containing cardiac glycosides should be dried at temperatures not exceeding 50°C, for otherwise there is a decrease in the active glycoside concentration. On the other hand temperatures of less than 40°C allow enzymes to break down active principles during the drying process; this is known as catabolism and is a natural process characteristic of drying tissues. Drying temperatures for the various drug plants are given in the pictorial section of this book.

An important economic statistic is the *drying ratio*, which expresses the proportion between the weight of a specific quantity of fresh plant parts and that of the resultant dried crude drug. This varies not only according to the type of drug but also according to the condition of the fresh plant. Medicinal plants harvested in dry regions or following a dry period naturally have a lower water content and therefore also lose less during the drying process. Fleshy plants have a higher drying ratio than those with little succulence. Of all plant parts bark has the lowest drying ratio, for example, in Oak bark *(Cortex quercus)* it is 3:1, which means that 3 kilograms of fresh bark yield 1 kilogram of the crude drug. Roots also have a low drying ratio, for instance, that of Cinquefoil root *(Radix tormentillae)* is 3:1, Restharrow root *(Radix ononidis)* 3:1, Valerian root *(Radix valerianae)* 4:1, *Inula helenium* root *(Radix helenii)* 4:1, and Deadly Nightshade root *(Radix belladonnae)* 5:1. As a rule the drying ratio of leaves and aerial parts is 4:1 — 6:1, and of flowers 6:1 — 8:1. The drying ratio of fleshy fruits is naturally far greater, for example, that of the Elderberry *(Fructus sambuci)* is 8:1, while Blueberry *(Fructus myrtilli)* is 10:1.

Dried drugs are stored according to the character and quantity of the drug in sacks or other containers or else left unpacked — Ergot Fungus *(Claviceps purpurea)* for example — in which case they are packed in bags just before shipment. Drugs which absorb moisture readily should be put in plastic containers, such as P.V.C. bags. Drugs containing volatile oils are an exception to this rule, as it is better to store them in layers of paper bags, cardboard containers or tins. Poisonous drugs must be dried separately and the containers in which they are packed must be well labelled to avoid any possibility of mix-ups.

Drugs, whether they are stored at home, in the pharmacy or in storerooms, must be kept in a dark and dry place at a temperature not exceeding 18°C, in airtight containers that limit their deterioration and contamination. In all drugs storage causes a gradual loss of efficacy for many active constituents deteriorate with the passage of time, even though this process may be very slow. For that reason drugs should be no more than two years old on the average. The British Pharmaceutical Codex (B.P.C.) gives standards for moisture content for all crude drugs which are official drugs in this country. Normally this is 18 per cent by weight as determined by the official loss or drying test. In the case of *Digitalis purpurea* the limit is only 8 per cent because of the highly active catabolic enzymes found in this crude drug. In such cases storage with a drying agent such as silica gel or calcium chloride might be advisable. If correctly stored some alkaloid-containing plants retain at least some of their potency for great periods of time. Interesting recent research by a group of British pharmacognosists has shown the presence of alkaloids in herbarium samples that are several centuries old.

PREPARING MEDICINES FROM PLANTS

The preparation of medicines from plants and the various forms of these extracts are the subject of a special branch of science known as Galenic pharmaceutics, or Galenism, after the famous Greek physician Claudius Galen (c. 131—200 AD). He was the first to record extensively preparations or extracts made from crude drugs.

Crude drugs, dried roots, herbs, leaves, flowers and fruits, for example, are still used today in preparing extracts from plants. Fresh plants are used only exceptionally. Crude drugs must be prepared before use, that is they must be cut or crushed to varying degrees of fineness, roughly about six, ranging from coarse particles to fine powder. These grades are determined with the aid of meshes (sieves) of varying sizes and are known as coarse, medium or fine powders.

The simplest medicines prepared from drugs are HERBAL TEAS, which may contain only one drug — such as Chamomile tea *(species chamomillae)* or Lime-blossom tea *(species tiliae)* — or a combination of two or more that complement each other to produce the desired tints or fragrance. These teas are widely used home remedies for the treatment of constipation and indigestion, for use as sedatives, diuretics and stomachics, and even simply for their pleasant taste as beverages. The various plants used to make up tea mixtures must be thoroughly mixed so that they are equally dispersed. The preparation of herbal teas is dealt with in the following chapter.

An EXTRACT is a prepared form of the crude drug using either water or alcohol; it is prepared as a liquid *(extracta fluida)*, thin *(extracta tenuia)*, thick *(extracta spissa)* or dry *(extracta sicca)* extract, according to the time allowed for evaporation and concentration after preparation. This requires professional training and special equipment, such as efficient pan or film evaporators, and is therefore difficult to do outside a pharmacy.

TINCTURES are generally extracts from drugs obtained by means of an alcoholic medium. They are prepared by pouring diluted alcohol over the drug, which is generally placed in a glass bottle, and shaking the mixture several times a day. After eight to ten days the medium is poured off and filtered so that the tincture is not cloudy. Tinctures, as well as extracts, are the basic preparations for making up medicines in a pharmacy. Unlike extracts, however, they can be prepared in the home, for the procedure is fairly simple. Tinctures are used primarily in the form of drops to treat digestive upsets and coughs, and externally in the treatment of wounds and as gargles.

Other, now no longer common, forms of medicines include AROMATIC WATERS and SYRUPS. AROMATIC WATERS *(aquae aromaticae)* are aqueous solutions of essential oils prepared either by adding slowly the essential oil, diluted with alcohol, to the water, or by distillation of the drug containing the respective volatile oil.

SYRUPS *(sirupi)* are drug extracts thickened with sugar. The preparation of syrups consists of two stages. First it is necessary to prepare an extract or tincture from the drug and this is then boiled together with sugar and thickened. Syrups are used primarily in the treatment of coughs and diseases of the upper respiratory passages.

For external application — compresses, douches, mouth-washes — drugs are almost always prepared by maceration, infusion or decoction.

A quite special form of application are *cataplasma* used as masks and poultices. Only finely powdered drugs are used for this form of treatment, the powder being mixed with milk or water and heated to a thick consistency. Vitamin concentrates or other skin nourishing substances may be added to the mixture. Before it is used the mixture must be cooled to about body temperature (not above 40°C) and then applied to the treated spot for twenty to forty minutes. If the drug to be used for the preparation of the poultice contains an essential oil the mixture should not be boiled. Facial masks prepared from Chamomile as well as other combinations of drugs or fresh plants are used for cosmetic purposes.

Fresh, undried plants are only used to a limited extent, mostly in the form of poultices. They are either ground or finely chopped and applied to the treated spot directly or wrapped in a cloth. This method is the most common in popular home treatment. The juice of fresh plants is used internally. Such a preparation cannot be stored, however, and must always be freshly made. To prevent spoiling a preserving agent such as alcohol or a distillate is added to the juice or else it can be boiled with sugar. Fresh juice is rarely employed without previous preparation. One of the most well-known preparations of fresh juice is syrup of Garlic, a popular home remedy for many ailments.

In conclusion it is necessary to stress the importance of observing rigid conditions of hygiene in the preparation of medicines. This is particularly necessary with preparations made with water or with low concentrations of alcohol as fungal, yeast and bacterial spores will grow in the nutritive plant extract. Teas and aqueous extracts must not be used after two to three days and are best freshly prepared for each occasion. Crude drugs are natural substances and are therefore heavily contaminated with spores of micro-organisms, a problem overcome in the pharmacy by using alcohol or by making an extract with a strong sugar solution (syrups), both techniques preventing the growth of yeast and fungal spores. The magnitude of the problem is evident from recent warnings in the British Pharmaceutical Press about contamination of crude plant drugs. Because alcohol is not available without a license, syrups may be prepared for home remedies or it is also possible to use a wine for the extraction in place of water if the preparation is not required for immediate use.

MAKING HERBAL TEAS

Only properly prepared teas contain the optimum quantity of active principles. To this end it is necessary to use the required quantity of the drug and water of the proper temperature for extraction of the active constituents.

First of all, a few words about how much of the drug should be used. It is wrong to believe that the greater the amount used in making the tea the better the effect. A high concentration of the active principles may have the very opposite effect to that desired by the patient and therefore it is not advisable to use more than the prescribed amount which, furthermore, years of practice have proved to be the most efficacious. For correct dosage it may prove helpful to remember that a rounded — not heaped — teaspoonful equals 1.5—2 grams and a tablespoonful about 5 grams of a herbal tea mixture. If instead of a tea mixture the crude drug is used as such, then 1 teaspoonful equals about 3 grams of flowers, 4—5 grams of leaves and 6—10 grams of roots, wood or fruits. If the prescribed dosage is for one cup of tea that means for 100—150 millilitres of liquid. Far more of the drug is used for baths and compresses — on the average about 150—400 grams (half that amount for children).

Drugs purchased for this purpose in the pharmacy have already been cut or crushed to a certain size, ranging from coarsely cut particles (about 6 millimetres in diameter), finely cut (3 millimetres) to coarsely crushed (2 millimetres). Drugs in finer form — coarse to fine powders — are not generally used. For home use in teas the coarser cut is recommended.

There are several methods of preparing medicinal teas and these may be classified according to the temperature of the water, the extracting medium, used to make them.

Lengthy steeping of the drug for several hours at normal temperatures (15—20° C) is called *maceration*. This method is used primarily in those cases where the drug is easily separated into its constituent elements in water.

Maceration at higher temperatures, as a rule 35—40° C but not more than 50° C, is called *digestion*. This method is used primarily for hard barks or woods which are difficult for water to penetrate.

If the drug is boiled for ten minutes or if boiling water is poured over it and allowed to stand for thirty minutes, the result is called a *decoction*.

The most common method of preparing a medicinal tea is as an *infusion*. The drug is placed in a pot and wetted with cold water and immediately afterwards boiling water is poured over it, then left to stand, covered with a lid for about fifteen minutes, after which the tea is poured off.

Sugar is generally not added to medicinal teas nor are fruit syrups unless so prescribed. They should be sipped slowly while warm, one or more times a day depending on the character of the illness and the type of tea. It should, however, be remembered that all crude drugs are poisonous to a greater or less extent and self-medication is not to be recommended without qualified advice. Acutely toxic plants are legally controlled and are only available on the prescription of a qualified physician. They therefore provide no hazard. There are nevertheless many crude drugs available from the pharmacy or drug store which could be dangerous if misused. Helpful advice on the properties, dosage and preparation of these herbs may be readily obtained from the local registered pharmacist.

CULTIVATING DRUG PLANTS

The cultivation of drug plants is a fairly recent branch of plant production that can be traced back to the monastery gardens of mediaeval times which produced drugs for the monasteries' medicinal needs. Commercial production of certain medicinally important plants, however, dates only from the second half of the nineteenth century, being directly linked with the growth of the pharmaceutical industry; in recent years this type of production has greatly increased. Cultivated predominantly as garden plants in the early twentieth century, herbs are now grown on a large scale as field crops harvested mechanically, in the same way as other common farm crops such as cereals and root vegetables, with machines specially adapted for the purpose.

At least 100 species of medicinal plants are currently cultivated in the temperate and subtropical regions, about thirty of them as large-scale field crops, for example Chamomile *(Matricaria chamomilla)*, Caraway *(Carum carvi)*, Valerian *(Valeriana officinalis)*, Opium Poppy *(Papaver somniferum)*, Peppermint *(Mentha × piperita)*, *Digitalis lanata*, Ergot Fungus *(Claviceps purpurea)*, Marsh Mallow *(Althaea officinalis)*, and Deadly Nightshade *(Atropa belladonna)*.

Unlike classic farm crops most medicinal plants grown on a commercial scale have only recently been introduced to cultivation. The majority, therefore, still exhibit the same characteristics as the wild plant, which often renders successful cultivation difficult — for example, the period of germination and ripening is not uniform. Cultivated plants require further breeding and selection to obtain higher yields, uniform germination, growth and maturation, as well as a higher concentration of the active principles. Large-scale cultivation also makes necessary the development of new mechanical aids, especially for harvesting. Otherwise the cultivation of medicinal plants is governed by the same principles as that of other crops.

Some drug plants such as Caraway *(Carum carvi)*, Fennel *(Foeniculum vulgare)* and Coriander *(Coriandrum sativum)* can be cultivated in the same way as cereals, others as root crops, for example Valerian *(Valeriana officinalis)*, *Digitalis lanata*, and Deadly Nightshade *(Atropa belladonna)*, and those grown for their aerial parts like forage crops — Peppermint *(Mentha × piperita)* and Common Balm *(Melissa officinalis)*, for example. It is always necessary to bear in mind, however, that the similarity in the techniques of cultivation is only of a general nature.

Successful cultivation of medicinal plants requires the same conditions as the successful cultivation of other crops, namely that each particular species is given the right soil and climate to suit its needs. This is of particular importance in the case of plants that are to be cultivated in areas other than that of their natural distribution. For instance, if heat-loving species are to be grown in more northerly regions it is necessary to select areas with the greatest similarity to their natural habitat. Insufficient heat must be counterbalanced by better quality soil, balanced nutrition and greater moisture. Sometimes the plants require increased protection against infectious diseases that do not occur in their native habitat. At the same time growers should try to breed new varieties with the same concentration of active constituents but better adapted for cultivation in areas climatically different from their natural habitat. In short, the yield and concentration of active principles in drug plants is markedly influenced by soil conditions and climate, as are all agricultural crops.

CLIMATE

It is difficult to determine the influence of climate, which comprises many factors such as temperature, rainfall, sunlight, air currents and altitude above sea level, on plants.

For example, its influence on the concentration of active principles contained in the organs of a plant is well known. Higher mean temperatures have a favourable effect on the formation of essential oils as, for example, in Fennel *(Foeniculum vulgare)*, White Horehound *(Marrubium vulgare)*, and Lavender *(Lavandula spica)*, but Chamomile *(Matricaria chamomilla)*, cultivated in warm subtropical regions does not exhibit any improvement in its therapeutic qualities. True, it has a high concentration of essential oil but often this oil lacks chamazulene, the constituent responsible for its anti-inflammatory action. On the other hand, Chamomile from the colder central European countries (Czechoslovakia, Hungary and Germany) has a high concentration of chamazulene. The reaction of alkaloid plants such as Henbane *(Hyoscyamus niger)*, Jimson Weed *(Datura stramonium)* and Deadly Nightshade *(Atropa belladonna)* to higher temperatures and increased sunlight is higher alkaloid production, whereas in low temperatures, with long periods of rain and cloudy weather, their alkaloid content decreases fairly rapidly. It has been proved that excessive moisture reduces the quantity of mucilages in Marsh Mallow *(Althaea officinalis)* and Common Mallow *(Malva silvestris)*. Autumn frosts lower the concentration of glycosides in the leaves of *Digitalis lanata*, often before they are harvested. Shade also reduces the quantity of active principles, for example, the amount of essential oil in Chamomile *(Matricaria chamomilla)*. The above examples are sufficient indication of the role climate plays in the quality of drug plants.

SOIL AND NUTRITION

The quantity and quality of the active constituents in medicinal plants are also determined by the type of soil in which they are grown, mainly its fertility, chemical, biological and physical characteristics as well as its nutritive value. Plants harvested for their roots, rhizomes or tubers cannot, for instance, be cultivated in heavy, clinging soil not only because of the difficulty of ploughing and cleaning but also because the concentration of active principles they produce when grown in such soil is lower.

This has been proved, for instance, in Rhubarb *(Rheum palmatum)*, Parsley *(Petroselinum crispum)*, Marsh Mallow *(Althaea officinalis)*, and Gentian *(Gentiana lutea)*. Xerophitic drug plants which thrive in hot, dry soils cannot be cultivated in damp soils nor water-loving ones in dry soils.

In alkaline or chalky soils *Digitalis lanata* not only gives higher yields but also a higher concentration of glycosides than in soils which are slightly acidic. *Digitalis purpurea*, on the other hand, does not tolerate calcium in the soil and has higher yields as well as a higher concentration of glycosides in acidic soils. Similarly, Chamomile *(Matricaria chamomilla)*, has greater yields and a higher content of essential oil when grown on soils rich in calcium.

Soils rich in nitrogenous substances increase the amount of active principles in alkaloidal plants as was determined, for instance, in Jimson Weed *(Datura stramonium)*, Deadly Nightshade *(Atropa belladonna)*, and Ergot Fungus *(Claviceps purpurea)*.

Experimental studies carried out to date have shown that even insufficient trace elements, such as manganese, zinc and magnesium, for example, lower the production of glycosides.

The yields and quality of drug plants can be greatly improved by fertilization — with potash fertilizers in the case of plants grown for their roots or rhizomes, phosphoric fertilizers in the case of those grown for their flowers and fruits, and nitrogen fertilizers in the case of those where the leaves and top parts are harvested.

There is much contrary information available on what influence soil fertilization has on the concentration of active principles in drug plants, but it is hoped that this will finally be established in the near future by properly conducted experiments. Of the artificial preparations for drug plant cultivation now on the market only one has shown significant positive results. This is chlorcholine chloride (CCC) which increases the concentration of alkaloids in ergot obtained by cultivation of Rye Ergot.

We hope this book fulfills its intended purpose of informing the general public about the present-day importance of medicinal plants, the active principles they contain, their collection, therapeutic effects, and methods of use. Though brief, we hope it will serve to convince the reader that drug plants are, and will long continue to be, important therapeutic agents when properly administered under the supervision or with the advice of a qualified physician.

Achillea millefolium L. Compositae

Milfoil, Yarrow

This is a perennial herb, flowering from June to September. It grows in abundance in meadows, hedgerows, woodland clearings and copses, by the wayside, in sandy and barren places and as a weed, from lowland to alpine elevations above the tree line. It is distributed over the temperate regions of Europe and western Asia, and north of the Arctic Circle it is found in the vicinity of man and his herds. It has also been introduced into North America, southern Australia and New Zealand.

The flowering top parts *(Herba millefolii)* are collected for the drug market. These are cut off several centimetres above the ground during the flowering period and either spread out to dry in thin layers or hung in bunches in a shaded and well-ventilated spot. The temperature in drying rooms must not exceed 40° C. The plant has an aromatic odour and bitter taste, and can cause dermatitis in sensitive persons. It has an essential oil content of up to 0.5 per cent, which among other substances contains chamazulene, which is therapeutically the most effective constituent. Flavones and tannins are also present. The drug stimulates the flow of gastric secretions and has a beneficial effect on the blood circulation. Its action is anti-inflammatory and is thought to check internal bleeding.

It is administered internally in the form of an infusion in gastric and digestive upsets, as a haemostatic in lung haemorrhage, kidney haemorrhage and excessive menstrual flow. Externally it is used in the treatment of rashes and as a gargle in inflammation of the gums.

This drug is not grown in cultivation, but as it has been found that Milfoil often lacks azulene it is recommended that varieties which are rich in chamazulene should be cultivated.

Flowering plant

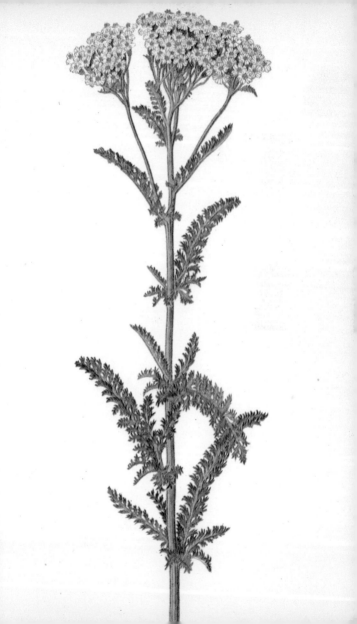

† *Aconitum napellus* L.

Ranunculaceae

Monkshood, Aconite

This perennial herb flowers in July and August. It has a sparse to fairly abundant distribution, often growing in large clumps, in pastures and meadows, in alder groves, beside streams, in ditches and beside mountain cottages at mountain (600—800 metres) to alpine elevations. Beside streams it is often found low down in the valleys. It is collected in the mountains of central Europe and as far north as Sweden. Related types, considered separate species by some authors, occur in Asia, from the Caucasus to the Far East.

The drug is obtained from young, daughter rhizomes (*Tuber aconiti*) collected after flowering from July to September. Very great care must be taken in collecting as the plant is extremely poisonous. Cleaned and halved or sliced rhizomes are dried rapidly at a temperature not exceeding 40° C. The drug is odourless and has a pungent taste. It should be kept in a dry place for moisture, like lengthy storage, decreases the efficacy of the active principles. The drug contains highly toxic, comparatively unstable alkaloids which easily change into far less efficient but equally poisonous products under the influence of water. The best known alkaloid is aconitine (one of the most violent poisons of the plant kingdom). The drug affects the central and peripheral nervous system, first as a stimulant and then as an analgesic.

The drug is no longer used as a medicament but only for the recovery of aconitine, one of the components of pharmaceutical specifics for the treatment of neuralgic and rheumatic pains and especially effective in certain cases of trigeminal neuralgia. It is applied externally in the form of an ointment in the treatment of rheumatism. Preparations from this plant may be prescribed only by a physician.

The drug is collected only in the wild.

1. *Rhizomes*
2. *Part of the flower stem*

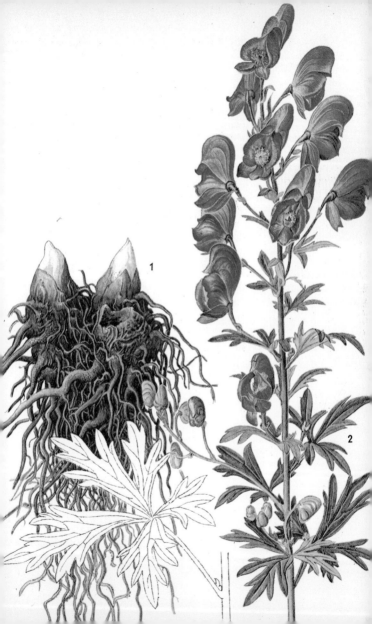

1

2

Acorus calamus L.

Sweet Flag

This is a perennial herb which flowers in June and July. It is fairly widely distributed and locally abundant, by the edges of ponds and slow-flowing waterways, in ditches and marshes, from lowland to mountain elevations. This plant is believed to be indigenous only in the area extending from northern India to Ceylon, the Himalayas and Assam. It spread throughout Europe from plants first cultivated in the Vienna botanical garden in 1576. European and certain east Asian and North American plants belong to the variety *calamus*, in eastern Asia the variety *spurius* is found and on the Atlantic coast of North America the variety *americanus*. The range of distribution may be described as circumpolar with the inclusion of those areas where it has evidently become established, and may be found growing wild in many parts of Europe.

The drug is obtained from the rootstock *(Radix calami aromatici)* collected in the autumn. This is cut into pieces 10—15 centimetres long and dried at a temperature not exceeding 40° C, either naturally or with artificial heat. The rootstock should not be peeled for this lowers its essential oil content. The drug has a distinct odour and pungent flavour. It contains 2—6 per cent of an essential oil. Bitter principles and tannins are also present. The drug stimulates digestion and metabolism, exerts a mild diuretic action and relieves flatulence.

It is used internally in powder, tincture, infusion and extract form — previously it was also candied — as an aromatic bitter principle to stimulate the appetite, and in digestive disturbances, colic, flatulence, and diarrhoea. The effect is produced by a whole group of substances. Externally the drug is used as a gargle to relieve sore throat and as a mildly stimulating agent in baths. A volatile oil, the composition and quantity of which differ according to whether the origin of the herb is European, Indian or Japanese, can also be isolated from the plant and is used in the food industry and in perfumery and cosmetic preparations as well as medicinally.

The drug is collected only in the wild.

1. *Flower*
2. *Rootstock*

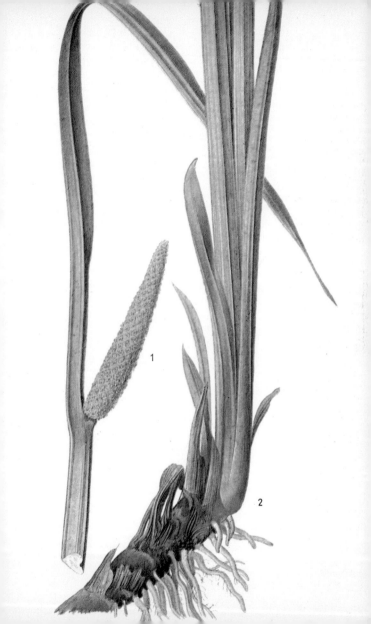

1

2

† *Adonis vernalis* L.

Ranunculaceae

Adonis

Adonis is a perennial herb, flowering in April and May, which is thinly distributed on alkaline soils on sun-warmed rocky slopes, dry grassy hills, in copses and pinewoods, from lowland to hilly country in the warmest climates. It occurs in south-western, central and eastern Europe across the Crimea to Siberia as far as the middle reaches of the Lena River. The range of distribution extends roughly along latitude 50° N, but is more southerly in central Europe and more northerly to the east.

The flower tops *(Herba adonidis vernalis)* are collected for the drug market at the end of April and in May. The stems are cut off several centimetres above the ground and dried best by natural heat in the shade or by artificial heat at temperatures not exceeding 50° C. The drug, which has a marked bitter taste, must not be brownish and should be stored in tightly stoppered jars so that it is kept dry. It contains toxic glycosides which stimulate cardiac activity. Unlike *Digitalis* glycosides, they do not accumulate in the heart muscle because the drug exerts a diuretic action and the active principles are eliminated in the urine.

It is used internally in the form of an infusion or tincture. Isolated glycosides in the form of drops are prepared only on prescription for the treatment of minor cardiac insufficiency or when necessary to alternate heart medicines in the case of long-term application. Medicines made from Adonis also alleviate accompanying nervous disorders.

The drug is collected mostly in the wild, its cultivation having been attempted only in isolated instances. Other, mainly annual, species of the genus *Adonis* contain similar medicinal substances but in much smaller quantities.

Flowering plant

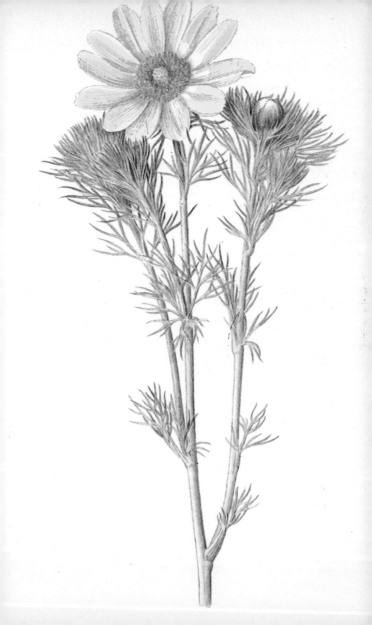

Aesculus hippocastanum L. Hippocastanaceae

Horse Chestnut, Buckeye

This tree, blooming in May and June, is indigenous to the hills of the Balkan Peninsula but it is also found in south-west Asia and the Himalayas. It is frequently cultivated from lowland to mountain elevations — although in the latter it does not bear fruit — in avenues and parks, and occasionally in the woods, at the margins of which it often becomes established in the wild. In Europe cultivation has extended its range as far as the northern areas.

The seeds *(Semen hippocastani)* and to a lesser degree the flowers *(Flos hippocastani)* and bark *(Cortex hippocastani)* are collected for the crude drug. Ripe seeds (chestnuts) are gathered in the autumn, pre-dried under good ventilation and then further dried at a temperature of up to 60° C. The flowers are collected in dry weather and dried in the shade at normal temperatures. The bark is peeled in the spring. The crude drug is odourless and has a bitter flavour. As yet the constituents are not thoroughly known, but they are principally triterpene saponins, flavones and coumarins. The therapeutic effect is believed to be due mainly to the saponin component; the coumarin aesculin is also being tested for its medicinal action. The therapeutically remarkable substance in the flowers is a flavonoid aglycone, and in the bark tannins.

The drug has an anti-inflammatory and anti-oedematous effect. It also has antispasmodic and anticoagulant properties, besides having a beneficial effect on sclerosis. Preparations from the seeds are an important medicament in the treatment of varicose veins and haemorrhoids. They are used internally in the form of drops or injections, externally as ointments and in baths. All preparations from Horse Chestnut are dispensed only on prescription by a physician.

The drug is not cultivated but collected only in the wild.

1. *Flowering branch*
2. *Seed (chestnut)*

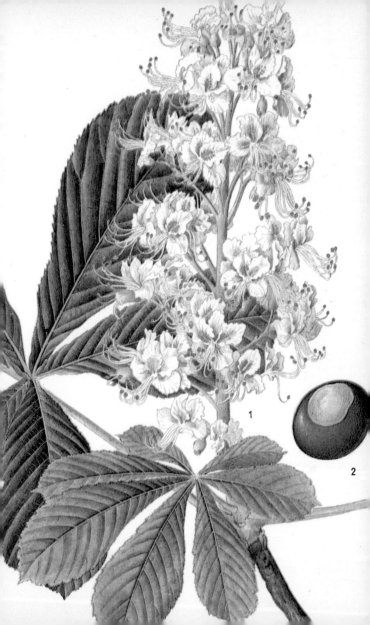

1

2

Agrimonia eupatoria L.

Rosaceae

Agrimony

This perennial herb, flowering from June to August, grows freely in pastures, copses and woodland clearings, in hedgerows and by the roadside, from lowland to submontane elevations. The range of distribution embraces northern, central and eastern Europe including the Caucasus. Sometimes the specific name *eupatoria* is used to describe all the various species — about ten — whose area of distribution is roughly the temperate zone of the Northern Hemisphere. Most of them probably contain active principles of the same quality as *A. eupatoria*.

For medicinal purposes the flowering tops *(Herba agrimoniae)* are collected before the seeds have formed from June to August. These are cut off several centimetres above the ground and dried in thin layers in a well-aired and shady place or in a drying room at a temperature not exceeding 45° C. The drug has a faintly aromatic odour and slightly bitter taste. It contains tannins, flavone dyes, traces of an essential oil undetermined precisely as yet, and bitter principles. It has astringent, anti-inflammatory and costive properties and regulates stomach as well as liver function, including that of the gall bladder.

It is used internally in the form of an infusion or as a component in herbal tea mixtures for its markedly beneficial effect on the digestive organs, mainly the liver, gall bladder, stomach and intestines. Externally it is used as a gargle in stomatitis, in the form of compresses in stubborn and chronic skin rashes, and as an aid in accelerating the healing of wounds.

The drug is collected mostly in the wild because cultivation is difficult owing to the poor germination of the seed.

1. *Fruit (receptacle)*
2. *Top part of stem with flowers*
3. *Leaf*

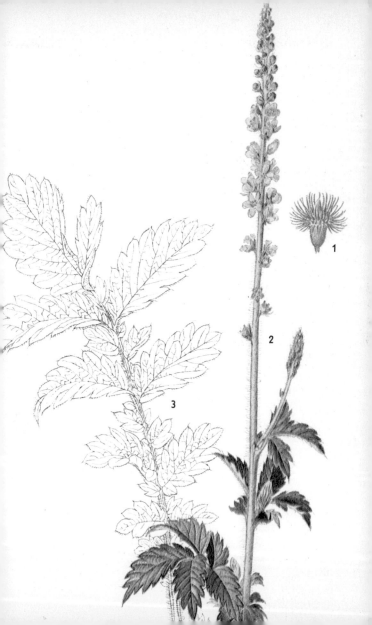

1

2

3

Allium cepa L.

Common Onion

This is a biennial as well as a perennial herb which flowers from June to August. It is a species which was originally grown from central Asia to south-west India. In the East and in Mediterranean regions it has been cultivated since ancient times. Today numerous cultivars are grown in most parts of the world; only in eastern Asia is *Allium fistulosum* L. cultivated in its place.

The Common Onion is one of the most widespread of vegetables and seasonings besides which it is also used for its medicinal properties. The part collected for medicinal purposes is the bulb *(Bulbus allii cepae)*. Only healthy and fully matured bulbs are collected and after removal of the leaves they are stored in sacks or on frames of wooden slats at a temperature of 3—5° C and in a relative humidity of 60 per cent. Dried Onion is very rarely used. The Onion has a marked pungent odour, causes the eyes to water and has a sweetish spicy taste. It contains substances which are chemically closely related to those of Garlic. Further constituents are flavonoid glycosides, pectin and glucokinins. These substances have an excellent germicidal effect, stimulate digestion and secretion of bile, and lower blood pressure.

Onion is used internally in various forms, in the same way as Garlic. It acts as a digestant, stimulates the appetite, lowers the blood sugar level and also has an expectorant action. It is also used for the expulsion of certain intestinal parasites. Externally it is used as a popular home remedy for acne.

Cultivation of the Onion was probably introduced into central Europe from Italy.

1. *Flowers*
2. *Bulb*

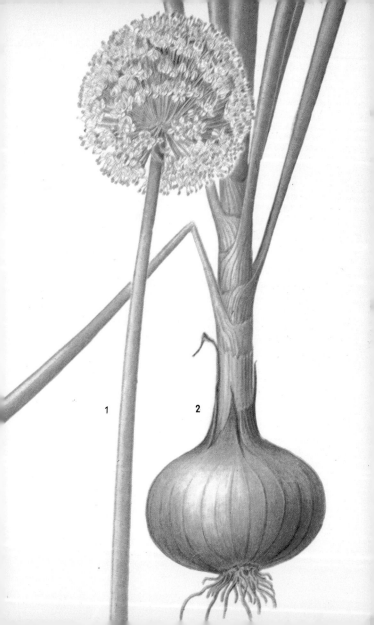

Allium sativum L.

Liliaceae

Garlic

This is a biennial and perennial herb flowering from June to August. A cultivar first grown in central Asia, it has been used for centuries past as a seasoning, vegetable and medicinal herb in the area extending from the Mediterranean to central Asia. Today it is practically worldwide in cultivation.

Fresh bulbs *(Bulbus allii sativi)* are the crude drug. They are harvested as soon as the leaves turn yellow — in July or August — for if this is left till later the bulbs break up into their individual cloves. When thoroughly dry the bulbs are stored in dry, frost-free premises. They have a distinctive pungent odour. Components include about 0.1 per cent of a malodorous essential oil with organic sulphur compounds, vitamins A, B and C and hormone-type substances. The drug acts as a carminative and vermicide, checks the growth of bacteria and fungi, increases the flow of bile and lowers blood pressure. External application, however, irritates the skin and may cause inflammation and blisters.

Garlic is used chiefly internally in the treatment of hypertension and arteriosclerosis, flatulence, intestinal catarrh of infectious aetiology, and for its anthelmintic action. It is also effective in treating bronchitis and the common cold. It is a popular seasoning for meat dishes, sausages and salamis, soups and gravies and is most widely used in the Mediterranean countries and in the East. It was most probably introduced into Europe from Italy by Roman colonizers.

1. *Flower*
2. *Bulb*
3. *Single clove*

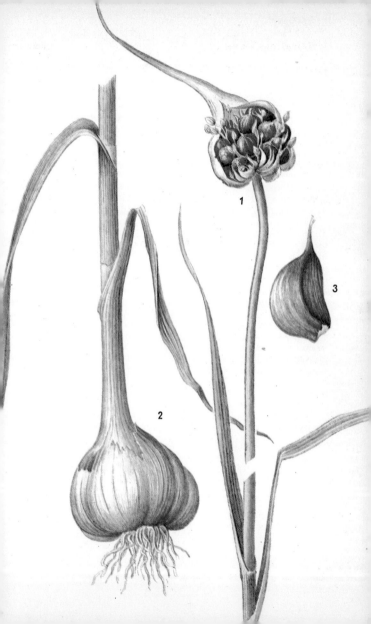

Althaea officinalis L.

Malvaceae

Marsh Mallow, Althea

This is a perennial herb flowering from July to September which has a scattered distribution in pastures and water meadows, in ditches and hedgerows, especially on salty soils, from lowland to hill elevations. It is found in central Europe, the Baltic countries, the areas bordering the rivers that feed the Black and Caspian Seas and in western Siberia all the way to central Asia.

The roots *(Radix althaeae)* and leaves *(Folium althaeae)* are the parts used for pharmaceutical purposes. Today these are mostly collected from cultivated plants. The roots are harvested in the autumn and stored in cellars or dugouts prior to peeling. Peeling removes the corky layer and part of the cortex, after which the roots are cut into smaller pieces or diced and dried at temperatures not exceeding 40° C. The leaves are collected before the flowering stage. The drug must not contain leaves attacked by rust or damaged by pests. The drug has a faint, distinctive odour and sweetish mucilaginous taste and contains about 10 per cent mucilage of unknown composition. In addition the roots contain other substances such as starch (about 38 per cent), sugar (about 10 per cent) and invert sugar. The leaves contain, in addition to mucilage, traces of an essential oil (0.02 per cent). The mucilages aid expectoration, soothe irritation of the mucous membrane and subdue inflammation.

The drug is used internally in macerated form — in cold water — and as a syrup or tea in the treatment of respiratory diseases when the mucous membrane is inflamed and irritated, to relieve a severe cough and asthma. In pediatrics it has an excellent effect in the treatment of diarrhoea and intestinal diseases.

The drug is obtained principally from cultivated plants grown in Belgium, Germany and the United States; its cultivation has been known from about the eighth century.

1. *Root*
2. *Top part of stalk with flowers*

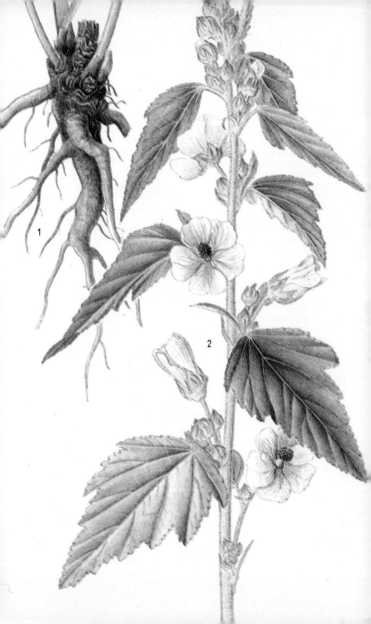

Anethum graveolens L.

Umbelliferae

Dill

Dill is an annual herb which flowers in July and August. It is probably indigenous to Iran and India, although Egypt and the Caucasus are also cited. It is cultivated in practically all parts of the world, and found growing wild and occasionally established in barren places, by the wayside, in hedges, fields and fallow land, in the vicinity of dwellings and on sandy river banks. In the Mediterranean region it has been known as a medicinal plant and stimulating condiment since ancient times. It was introduced into central Europe by Roman colonizers.

The parts used in pharmaceutics and the food industry are the fresh leaves *(Folium anethi)* or flowering tops *(Herba anethi)*. Dried Dill is not used as a drug. The odour is reminiscent of Caraway, the taste being sharp and sweetish at first, then distinctively spicy. Up to 1.5 per cent of an essential oil is found in the leaves and flowering stems and up to 4 per cent in the fruits or seeds. The oil yielded by the fruits contains primarily carvone, limonene and other substances. This essential oil has disinfectant and antispasmodic properties, relieves flatulence and promotes lactation.

Nowadays, Dill is scarcely used at all for medicinal purposes. Its principal use is as a condiment in sauces and salads, and in flavouring potatoes and pickled vegetables and fruits, where its preserving (phytoncidic) properties are useful. Dill seed is used in making herb butter, soup flavourings and other foods and dishes. The essential oils obtained from the fruits and leaves have similar uses.

Dill is widely cultivated as a herb, particularly in the Oregon and Ohio areas of the United States where the plant is grown chiefly for the isolation of its essential oils.

1. *Flowering and seed heads*
2. *Detail of a flower*
3. *Detail of a fruit*

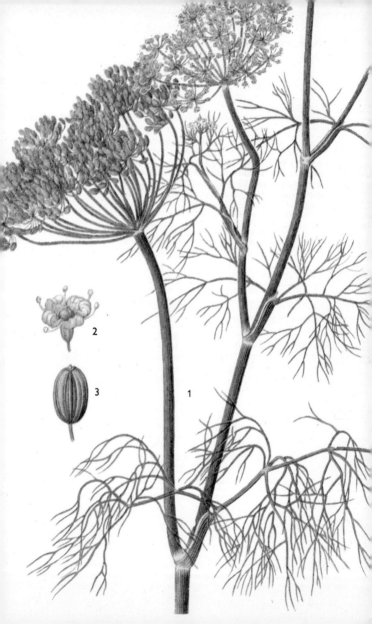

Anisum vulgare GAERTN.
(Pimpinella anisum L.)

Umbelliferae

Anise

This annual herb, flowering in July and August, is most probably indigenous to the eastern Mediterranean where it has been cultivated for centuries as a medicinal plant and flavouring. Sometimes it is found growing wild in rubbish dumps and barren places, but only temporarily.

The part collected for the drug market is the fruit *(Fructus anisi vulgaris)*. The seed heads are cut when they begin to turn yellow and near maturation. They are then tied into bunches and threshed after the fruit has ripened fully. The latter is then cleaned and dried, best of all by natural heat. The crude drug is very aromatic and has a sweetish flavour. The fruits contain about 3 per cent of an essential oil of which the principal constituents are anethole (80—90 per cent), methylchavicol and other substances. The essential oil stimulates gland secretion, has an antispasmodic and carminative action, and diminishes the desire to cough.

Internally it is used in the form of an infusion in gastric and intestinal disorders, painful spasms of the digestive tract (especially in children), to stimulate the appetite, relieve flatulence and cough and stimulate the secretion of the mammary glands. In addition to its use in pharmacy it is a good, tasty and aromatic ingredient employed by the food industry as a flavouring agent.

Anise is grown in the Mediterranean, the USSR, Belgium, Germany, Czechoslovakia, India, Japan, Central America and Chile. It is the oldest spice of the Umbelliferae family.

1. *Inflorescence*
2. *Detail of fruit*
3. *Detail of a single flower*
4. *Leaf*

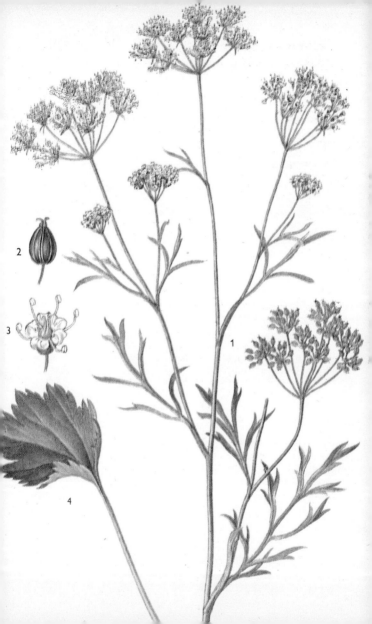

Anthemis nobilis L.
Compositae
(Chamaemelum nobile (L.) ALL.*)*

Chamomile

A perennial herb flowering from June to September, Chamomile is indigenous in the area from western Europe to Italy where it grows in pastures, on rocks and alongside walls. It is cultivated in numerous European countries and in some places may be found growing wild as an escape.

The part of the plant collected for pharmaceutical purposes is the inflorescence *(Flos chamomillae romanae)*, that is, the flower heads without the stalk. These are collected just at the beginning of the flowering stage, in dry, sunny weather from June to August. They should be dried as rapidly as possible in a well-ventilated place, preferably by natural heat; if in a drying room, then very carefully at temperatures not exceeding 35° C. The crude drug is aromatic and has a spicy bitter taste. If properly dried the drug remains white and does not turn yellow. It contains 1—5 per cent of an essential oil, flavonoid glycosides, bitter principles and other substances. It has an anti-inflammatory effect, acts as a mild disinfectant and alleviates spasms.

It is used internally mostly in the form of an infusion and in herbal teas administered in digestive disorders accompanied by cramps, and to alleviate menstrual pains. Externally it is applied in compresses on wounds, burns and swellings in the same way as the drug from *Flos chamomillae vulgaris*. The flower heads also yield a volatile oil used primarily in the manufacture of cosmetic preparations.

The drug is obtained from cultivated plants — chiefly from the cultivar Ligulosa in which all the flowers in the anthodium are tongue-shaped. Chief producers of the 'Roman chamomile' are England, Belgium, France and Germany, where it has been cultivated in the latter country since the sixteenth century.

Flowering plant

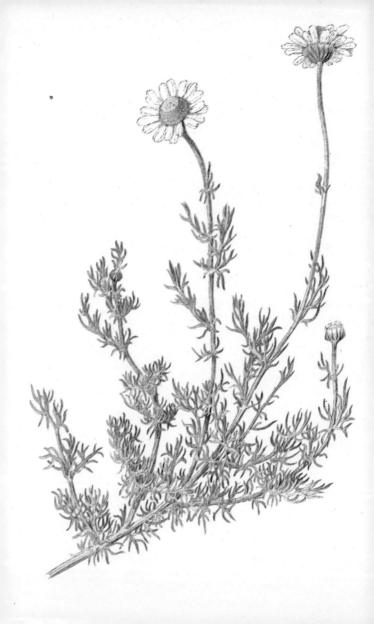

Archangelica officinalis (MOENCH) HOFFM.

Angelica   Umbelliferae

This is a biennial as well as a perennial herb which flowers from June to August and has a scattered distribution in damp meadows and thickets, in gullies and beside forest streams, at foothill to subalpine elevations. It is distributed in the temperate regions of Europe and Siberia from Greenland and Iceland to Kamchatka and the Aleutians, south to the Baikal, Altai and the Himalayas.

The drug is obtained from the roots *(Radix angelicae)* and fruit *(Fructus angelicae)*. The roots of cultivated plants in their second year of growth are principally collected. After harvesting and washing the roots are sliced and left to dry naturally, this being the best method. When dried by artificial heat the temperature must not exceed 45° C. The fruits are collected in August and September when ripe, left to dry thoroughly and then threshed and graded. The crude drug has an agreeable aromatic scent and spicy flavour. It must be kept in a dry place. Important centres of cultivation are Germany, France and the Netherlands, but the oldest is Scandinavia, where the plant has been grown since the twelfth century. The drug contains an essential oil; up to 1 per cent is obtained from the root, up to 1.5 per cent from the fruit. In small doses it stimulates the flow of gastric secretions and acts as an intestinal anodyne. In large doses, however, it has an undesirable effect on the central nervous system. Handling the drug may cause an allergic rash and irritation of the skin in some people.

The drug is employed in the form of an infusion or tincture, and in herbal tea mixtures in disorders of the digestive tract, to stimulate a poor appetite, and to relieve flatulence. The drug yields a volatile oil that is poisonous in large doses. Roots, seeds, stems and oil are also used in the food industry—as seasoning, to flavour liqueurs, and in crystalized form as a decoration, and in the manufacture of cosmetic preparations.

Angelica is cultivated in some European countries (var. *sativa*) and is sometimes found growing wild.

1. *Inflorescence*
2. *Flower*
3. *Root*

72

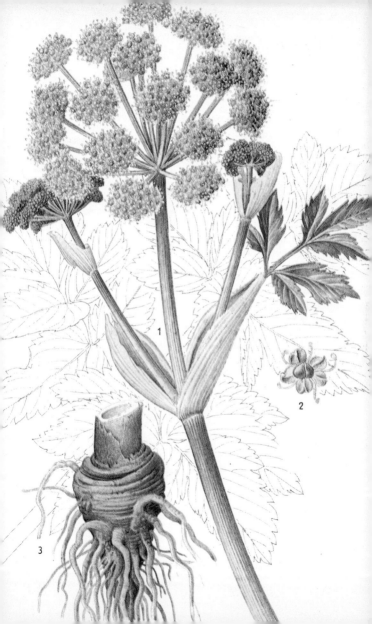

Arctostaphylos uva-ursi (L.) SPRENG.   Ericaceae

Bearberry

This shrub, flowering from April to June, is found scattered or in large clumps as undergrowth in thick woodland and juniper thickets and in rock hollows under snow in winter, at mountain to alpine elevations. Its range of distribution covers the arctic and temperate zone of the Northern Hemisphere, with the exception of the north of France, Belgium and the Netherlands where it does not occur at all. The southern boundaries of its range are the Mediterranean, the Altai and California. It is an age-old drug plant of the northern regions — there are records of its use dating from the twelfth century — but in central Europe physicians did not begin to use it until the eighteenth century.

The active principles are concentrated mainly in the leaves *(Folium uvae-ursi)* which are gathered by stripping from April to September, then dried in the shade in a well-ventilated spot. The drying process poses no problems, although some of the leaves turn brown and must be removed. The drug is odourless, slightly bitter and astringent on the tongue at first, with a sweetish aftertaste. It contains glycosides arbutin and methylarbutin and a fairly large amount of tannins. It is used medicinally for its diuretic and disinfectant properties. It is believed that the effective disinfectant component is a decomposition product of the glycosides.

Internally, it is best taken as an extract in cold water or else in the form of tea in the treatment of chronic inflammation of the urinary passages. It makes the urine turn dark. Use of the drug requires careful examination and must not be undertaken without the advice of a physician, as excessive dosing and long-term use may cause chronic impairment of the liver or, especially in children, the abundance of tannins may cause constipation and vomiting.

The drug is not cultivated but gathered only in the wild. The chief source of supply is the USSR.

1. *Flowering branch*
2. *Branch with fruits*

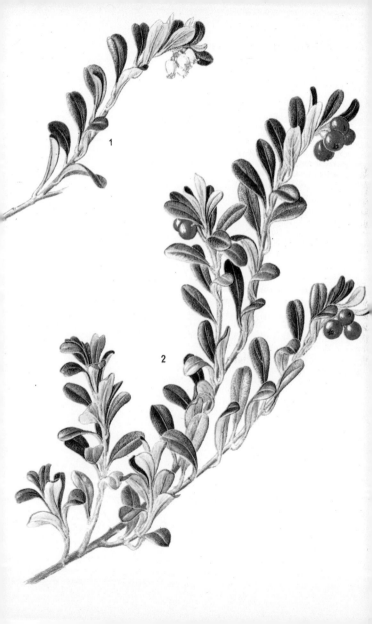

Armoracia rusticana GAERTN., MEY. *et* SCHERB.
(A. lapathifolia GILIB.*)*

Cruciferae

Horseradish

Horseradish is a perennial herb which flowers from May to July. It is indigenous only in the lowland areas and alongside the brooks and rivers of south-eastern Europe to western Asia, although it is often found growing wild in other regions near water and in damp thickets and on wasteland; in mountain areas sometimes even at elevations of 2000 metres. Horseradish has been cultivated in central Europe since the twelfth century, probably first of all by the Slavs, who already knew the herb in their original east-European home. It is now cultivated in Europe, North America, Chile, Japan and New Zealand.

Use is made of the fresh root *(Radix armoraciae)*, gathered in the autumn. It contains about 0.05 per cent of mustard oil and vitamin C. The mustard oil irritates the skin and causes blisters. In small doses it stimulates the function of the gastro-intestinal tract and dispels mucus, in large doses it may damage the lining of the stomach and the intestines.

Horseradish is used internally either grated or as a syrup in bronchial catarrh and to relieve 'spring tiredness', externally as a plaster to relieve rheumatic pains. Formerly it was used to treat inflammation of the kidneys and urinary bladder, and wounds that took a long time to heal. Some medicinal preparations countain bound mustard oil which is liberated after being taken internally; these are used in the treatment of infection and irritation of the urinary passages. Horseradish is a well-known condiment served grated with meat, sausages and salamis, and in cooking for sauces, meat and fish dishes. It is also used to flavour pickles and mustard.

1. *Root*
2. *Top part of a plant with flowers*

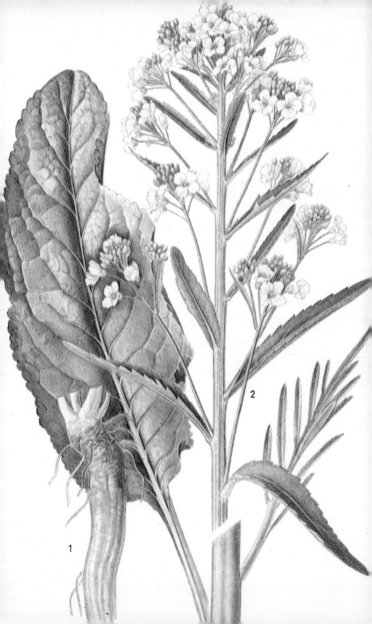

1

2

Artemisia abrotanum L.

Compositae

Southernwood, Lad's Love

This semi-shrub flowers from July to October; its native origin is unknown. The range of distribution extends from the Middle East to the Western Mediterranean, and in North America, where it was introduced. Southernwood is now found growing wild, having become established in the warmer regions.

The aerial parts *(Herba abrotani)* are collected for the drug market; they are cut off several centimetres above the ground from July to September during the flowering period. They are then spread out in thin layers and dried, without being turned, best of all in natural heat in the shade. The drug has a strong pungent odour and marked bitter taste. It contains an essential oil that has not been investigated thoroughly as yet, bitter principles, tannins and other substances. The bitter principles and certain constituents of the oil have a stimulating action on the gastric function. A mild antispasmodic and tonic effect has also been noted.

Internally, it is used as an infusion, sometimes also as a component of herbal tea mixtures in gastric disorders; externally, it is used as an aromatic ingredient of tonic bathwater preparations and as a poultice-type preparation applied to frostbite. Southernwood is sometimes used as a kitchen herb.

The drug is cultivated — in Germany, for example — but is now little in demand for medicinal purposes. It has been cultivated in Germany since the ninth or tenth century and also in various other parts of northern, central and eastern Europe, primarily in country gardens as an aromatic kitchen herb, and medicinal plant. In Mediterranean countries Southernwood has been known as a drug plant since ancient times.

Flowering shoot

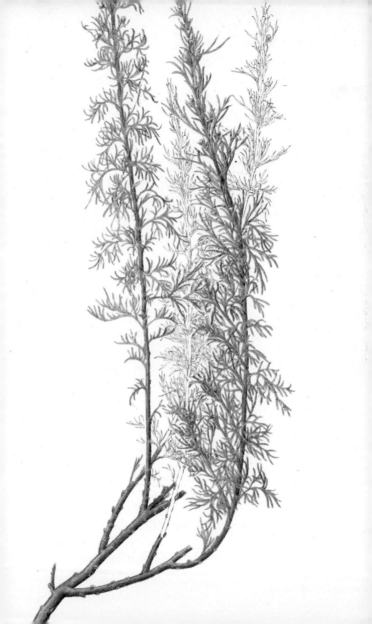

Artemisia absinthium L.

Compositae

Wormwood

This is a perennial herb or semi-shrub, flowering from June to September, which has a scattered, sometimes abundant, distribution on rocky hillsides, in pastures, along road verges, near dwellings and in waste places from lowland to foothill elevations. It became widespread in many parts of Europe centuries ago and now grows in practically all the temperate regions of Eurasia and Mediterranean countries, although it is not found in Greece and the Levant; it has been introduced to North and South America and New Zealand. It is believed to be indigenous probably only to some parts of the eastern Mediterranean.

Of importance for the drug market are the aerial parts *(Herba absinthii)*, collected during the flowering stage from June to August. The leaves and flowering shoots are spread out in thin layers or else tied in bunches and hung up to dry. Drying should take place in the shade in a well-ventilated spot or at a temperature not exceeding 40° C. The drug has a distinctive, very pungent odour and is aromatic and very bitter to the taste. It contains up to 0.5 per cent of an essential oil which increases the flow of bile and stimulates the appetite. Excessive use, however, is harmful for thujone, a constituent of the oil is toxic and causes inflammation, convulsions and intoxication.

The drug is administered internally in the form of an infusion or as an aromatic bitter preparation promoting digestion, and in gastric diseases. It must not be taken during pregnancy. An essential oil used to flavour bitter liqueurs, wines and aperitifs is also recovered from the herb; taken in excess, however, these drinks cause chronic poisoning and degeneration of the central nervous system.

The drug is both cultivated and gathered wild.

1. *Flowering shoot*
2. *Detail of a leaf*

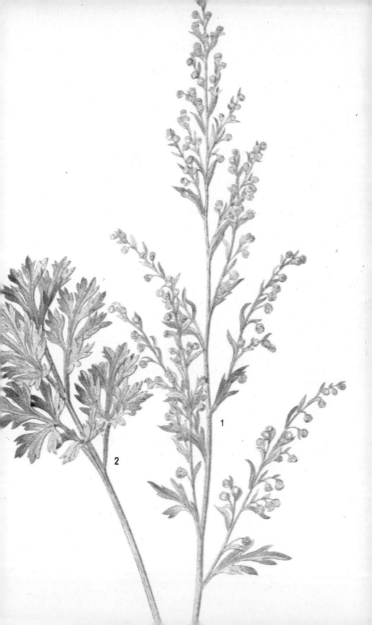

Artemisia dracunculus L. Compositae

Tarragon

Tarragon is a perennial herb or semi-shrub, flowering from July to October, with a scattered, sometimes locally abundant, distribution chiefly alongside rivers and streams in the central, southern and eastern regions of European Russia, Siberia, Mongolia and northern China, and in North America from the·west coast east as far as Colorado and Texas. It is cultivated chiefly in western Europe, in some places also in central Europe, primarily in the warmer, drier climates. It rarely grows wild, however.

The aerial parts *(Herba dracunculi)* minus the thicker stems, are collected for medicinal purposes at the beginning of the flowering stage in June and July. These are spread out in thin layers or hung up in bunches to dry in natural heat without unnecessary turning, or in drying rooms by artificial heat at temperatures not exceeding 40° C. The drug has an unpleasant odour and bitter aromatic taste. It contains 0.25—0.8 per cent of an essential oil. In addition to the oil Tarragon contains bitter principles and tannins. The presence of glycosides of the coumarin type has also been ascertained. Like the other types of Wormwood this one exerts a stimulating action on the digestive system, promoting the flow of digestive secretions and bile. Other effects are non-specific.

It is taken in the form of an infusion to stimulate the appetite, in the treatment of gastric and intestinal catarrh and intestinal parasite infestations, and also as a mild diuretic. Its use is prohibited in pregnancy. Both the fresh leaves and the oil are used in the food industry, as an aromatic in making tarragon vinegar and tarragon mustard, in soup seasonings, in the canning industry and, in minute quantities, also in perfumery.

The drug is obtained from cultivated plants. Most in demand on the market is German Tarragon, which is also, rather confusingly, known as French Tarragon.

Flowering shoot

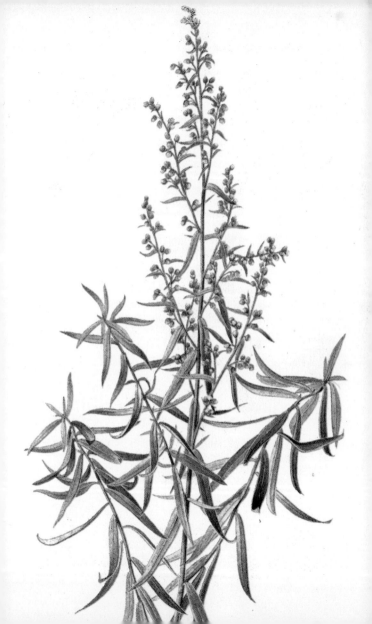

† *Atropa belladonna* L.

Solanaceae

Belladonna, Deadly Nightshade

This is a perennial herb, flowering from June to August, with a scattered distribution in shady deciduous forests — especially on the margins of beechwoods — in clearings and pastures, from hilly country to subalpine elevations. It is cultivated but often grows wild in central and southern Europe. Other species of this plant are found further east. It was probably introduced into the British Isles and Denmark as well as North America.

The part used for the extraction of the active principles is the root *(Radix belladonnae)*, less frequently the leaves *(Folium belladonnae)* or shoots *(Herba belladonnae)*. The roots of two-year plants are ploughed up at the end of October. After cleaning the thicker roots are cut in half and dried with artificial heat at temperatures not exceeding 70° C. Leaves and shoots are also dried rapidly and packed immediately as they are hygroscopic and readily turn black. The drug is odourless and has a bitter taste. As it is extremely poisonous collectors must take care in gathering and handling the plant, to protect the hands and especially the eyes. The drugs, like those of Henbane and Jimson Weed, contain tropane alkaloids, the leaves about 0.5 per cent and the roots up to 1.5 per cent. They affect the autonomic nervous system, decrease secretion of the salivary glands, inhibit gastric secretion and relax smooth muscle.

Today use is made of the pure alkaloids in various pharmaceutical specifics or stabilized extracts in the treatment of various diseases caused by disorders of the nervous centres, or which involve the functioning of smooth muscle. They are used as antispasmodics and anodynes, in relieving acute inflammation and colic, in neurology and ophthalmology, and for the treatment of complaints such as Parkinson's Disease.

The drug is gathered wild and cultivated. It is grown chiefly in eastern Europe — in Bulgaria and also in Hungary and Germany — in the form of cultivars with a high alkaloid content.

1. *Flower stem*
2. *Fruit*
3. *Root*

84

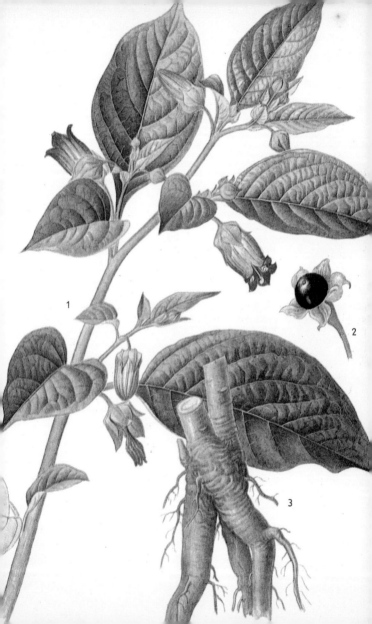

Betula verrucosa EHRH. *(B. pendula* ROTH*)*

Silver Birch

This is a tree, flowering in April and May, which grows abundantly in open deciduous and coniferous forests as admixture and undergrowth, in clearings, on slopes and rocky hillsides, often with a ground cover of heath, from lowland to mountain elevations. The range of distribution embraces Europe, the Middle East and western Siberia, south to the Altai and east to about longitude 100° E. It is generally found on acid, sandy-loamy to sandy, stony and peaty soils.

The parts collected for medicinal purposes are young spring leaves *(Folium betulae)* while they are still slightly sticky. These are dried in the shade or by artificial heat at temperatures not exceeding 45° C. The drug has a faintly aromatic, disagreeable odour and bitter taste. It contains saponins, some essential oil, resin, tannins and flavones. Young leaves also contain vitamin C. The drug has a diuretic and disinfectant action but does not irritate the kidneys. It also stimulates the sweat glands.

It is used internally as an infusion in diseases where the treatment requires increased excretion of urine to rid the body of harmful substances, such as diseases of the kidneys and urinary organs, rheumatism, gout and dropsy. The drug is therefore often used in urological herbal teas. Externally, it is used as a bath preparation. The bark and wood serve for the extraction of a tar containing cresol, traces of phenol and sulphur compounds. It has an antiparasitic action but is mildly irritating to the skin. 'Birch juice' is gathered in spring by tapping the tree trunks and is used as an additive in perfumery. Birch oil, also used in perfumery, is recovered from the young buds in quantities of 3.5 to 8 per cent, mainly in the United States.

The drug is not cultivated but gathered only in the wild.

1. *Branch with male and female catkins*
2. *Branch with male catkins*

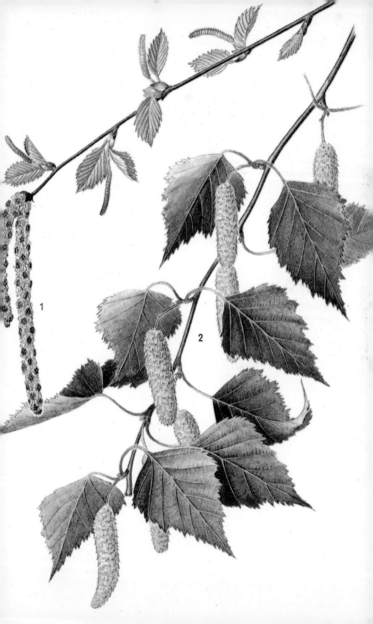

1

2

Borago officinalis L.

Borage

This is an annual herb flowering from May to September. It is most probably indigenous only to the western Mediterranean area, although some authorities think it is also native to the Middle East. Its cultivation was introduced by the Arabs in southern Spain in the early Middle Ages. It is grown in many parts of Europe, western Asia and North America, often growing wild in barren places, on compost heaps and on river banks, and occasionally in the Alps.

The aerial parts *(Herba boraginis)* are collected for medicinal purposes at the beginning of the flowering period from June to September and dried in the shade in thin layers. The drug has an odour reminiscent of Cucumber and a pleasant, pungent taste. It contains mucilages, saponins, tannins and other substances and has a mild diuretic, anti-inflammatory and cooling action. The effect, however, is non-specific.

The drug is used internally in the form of an infusion in inflammation of the urinary passages, rheumatism and heart diseases accompanied by oedema. Its main field of application is as a home remedy, having generally gone out of use in medicine. The fresh tops are prepared with Dill as a salad or as seasoning for salads.

The herb is gathered wild and also cultivated for home use.

Flowering top

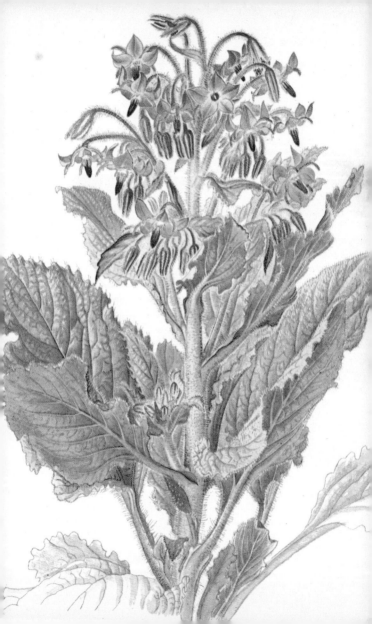

Brassica nigra (L.) KOCH

Cruciferae

Black Mustard

This annual herb flowers from May to October, and is most probably indigenous to the eastern Mediterranean or, according to some authors, from south-west Europe to central Asia. Cultivation has caused it to spread throughout the world, and it is now found both wild and established. It grows thinly — sometimes, however, in large numbers — on waste ground at the roadside, on riverbanks and in coastal scrub from lowland to hilly country, frequently on soil that is flooded at times.

The active principles are contained in the seed *(Semen sinapis nigrae)*. The plants are harvested as soon as the fruits are coloured yellow-brown, after which they are tied into bunches, left to ripen and then threshed and cleaned. The drug is odourless, has an oily taste and causes a sharp burning sensation on the tongue. In the presence of moisture the seeds yield a volatile oil which is extremely irritating to the eyes, stimulating the formation of tears. The seeds contain mustard glycosides, which upon hydrolysis yield volatile oil of mustard, about 30 per cent oil, proteins and other substances. The volatile oil is extremely irritating to the skin and mucous membranes. In small doses, however, it promotes gastric secretion and stimulates the appetite.

Medicinally, it is used in the preparation of irritant poultices and plasters for the treatment of rheumatism, acute inflammation of the respiratory passages and to improve the blood supply to deep-seated organs. If applied for too long, however, such a plaster may cause irritation and blistering of the skin. The seed was formerly used for the extraction of a volatile oil which is now obtained by synthetic means. Seeds of the White Mustard *(Sinapis alba)* are now used more frequently for the same purpose and also in the food industry.

The drug is obtained only from cultivated plants. Black Mustard is grown chiefly in the Netherlands, Italy and other Mediterranean countries as well as in North America.

1. *Flowering plant*
2. *Seed*
3. *Fruit*

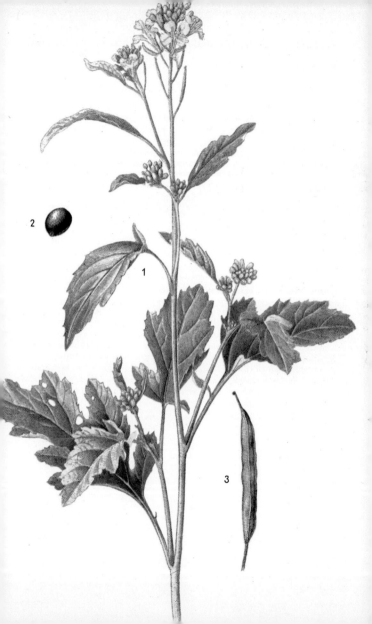

Capsicum annuum L.

Pepper

This is an annual to biennial herb, flowering from June to September. The types with small berries, believed to be the forerunners of the cultivated Red Pepper, grow in subtropical and tropical areas from the southern United States to the northern parts of South America. *Capsicum* is cultivated in warm regions throughout the world. It often grows wild but only transiently. The first peppers were introduced into Spain by Christopher Columbus and its cultivation in central Europe stems from the Mediterranean countries via the Balkan Peninsula. It was reintroduced into some countries of South America by European colonizers.

The part of the plant used for the extraction of the active principles is the fruit *(Fructus capsici)* of hot, small-fruited cultivars; these contain the greatest amount of capsaicin. The ripe fruits are dried slowly in a shady, well-ventilated spot. The drug has a characteristically spicy taste and causes a sharp, burning sensation on the tongue. It contains up to 2 per cent of capsaicin, classed as an alkaloid by most authorities, flavonoid glycosides, up to 0.2 per cent of vitamin C and traces of an essential oil of unknown composition. Capsaicin irritates and reddens the skin. In small doses it stimulates gastric secretion.

Capsicum is only rarely used as a drug and then in powder or tincture form, mainly to stimulate the flow of digestive secretions to promote gastric function. It is used more frequently for external application — in the form of ointments, liniments and plasters — in the treatment of rheumatism and arthritis. Its chief use, however, is as a condiment — sweet or hot pepper, cayenne pepper and chillies — or as a vegetable. The type used as a vegetable contains hardly any capsaicin but has a high vitamin content. Growers cultivate many different varieties.

1. *Part of a flowering plant*
2. *Fruit*

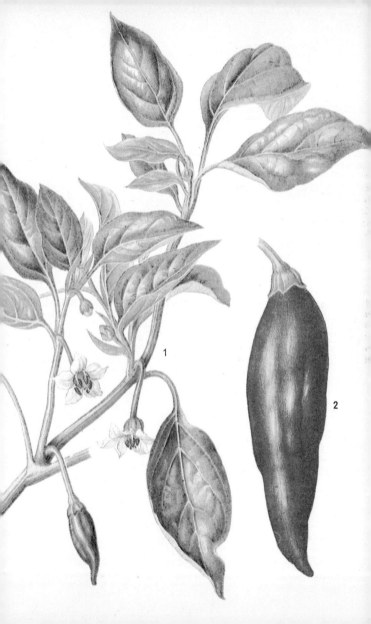

Carum carvi L.

Caraway

This annual herb flowers from May to July and grows in abundance in fields and meadows, at the edges of fields and roadsides and on waste ground from lowland to mountain elevations. The range of distribution extends from the arctic and temperate regions of Eurasia south to the Mediterranean, northern Iran, the Himalayas and Mongolia. In Africa it grows only in Morocco and it is not found at all in central and southern Italy, Greece or Asia Minor.

The drug is obtained from the fruit *(Fructus carvi)*. The harvesting of this plant, which is commonly cultivated for medicinal as well as culinary purposes, is very similar to the harvesting of grain. Caraway for both the food and pharmaceutical industries requires the same treatment and storage. The drug has the typical odour of Caraway and a sharp spicy taste. It contains 3—8 per cent of an essential oil. Caraway relieves flatulence, stimulates the function of the digestive organs and relaxes spasms of the smooth muscle. Its effect is similar to that of such related plants as Fennel and Anise.

It is used in various forms as a carminative and antispasmodic, as a tonic and in the treatment of digestive disorders, chiefly in pediatrics, in combination with other drugs such as Chamomile. Its use in herbal teas to relieve chest colds, to stimulate the mammary glands and to increase lactation in nursing mothers has also been known. Caraway is also used frequently in veterinary medicine. First and foremost, however, it is used by the food industry as a flavouring on bread and rolls, in cheeses, in cooking red beets, cabbage and potatoes, and in soups and sauces. Caraway oil is isolated from the fruit.

Caraway is cultivated chiefly in Europe, primarily in the Netherlands and the USSR, followed by Hungary, Germany and Czechoslovakia. It often grows wild.

1. *Inflorescences*
2. *Fruits*
3. *Detail of fruit*

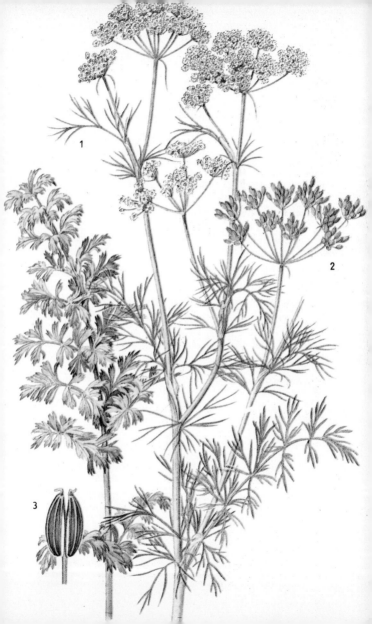

Centaurium minus MOENCH
(C. umbellatum GILIB.,
Erythraea centaurium PERS. *)*

Centaury

This is an annual as well as a biennial herb flowering from July to September, which has a scattered, sometimes abundant distribution on dry slopes, in meadows and forest clearings, and at the edges of fields and roadsides, from lowland to mountain elevations. It is distributed throughout most of Europe, from the Caucusus and Asia Minor across Iran to western Siberia. It has also been introduced into North America.

The active principle is extracted from the flowering tops *(Herba centaurii)*, the plants being cut off several centimetres above the ground in July and August. These are dried in the shade or at a temperature not exceeding 45° C. The drug is odourless and has a bitter taste. It contains glycosidic bitter principles and their decomposition products; these are the same type as those found in *Gentiana* species. The bitter principles increase the flow of gastric secretions, thereby improving digestion.

The drug is used internally in the form of an infusion, but preferably as a tincture, taken before meals, to stimulate the appetite and to aid digestion; it is also used in liver disorders coupled with decreased bile secretion. It is the principal constituent of the bitter gastric tincture *Tinctura amara* and various gastric herbal teas. It is also used in the production of certain bitter herb liqueurs.

The drug is gathered only in the wild, but attempts at semi-culture — cultivating the herb in natural localities — have, however, been successful. The drug has been known since the time of Dioscorides in the first century AD.

Flowering plant

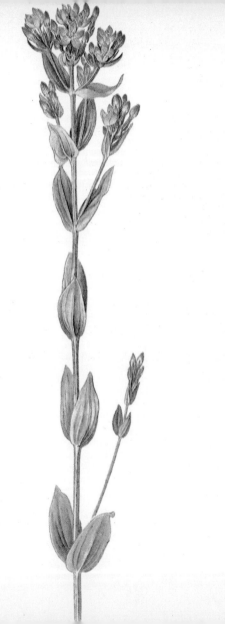

Cetraria islandica (L.) ACH.

Parmeliaceae

Iceland Moss

This is a lichen with a scaly, branched, erect thallus, coloured brown or greenish-brown when moist. It grows abundantly, often in large clumps, on the dry soil of mountain peaks and in the northern tundra from lowland to mountain elevations. Its range of distribution embraces the arctic and temperate regions of the Northern Hemisphere.

The part containing the active principle is the thallus, which is collected during dry weather from spring to autumn. When it has been cleaned of extraneous matter such as moss, it is dried rapidly by natural heat in a well-ventilated spot or in drying rooms by artificial heat at a temperature not exceeding 45° C. The crude drug is stiff when dry and produces a rustling sound; it has a bitter, mucilaginous taste. It contains mucilages, lichen acids and lichen starches. The content of mucilage and anti-bacterial substances has a beneficial effect in the treatment of respiratory diseases, including some types of tuberculosis.

The drug is used internally in the form of an infusion or in herbal teas in the treatment of catarrh of the upper respiratory passages, and as a supplementary medicine in certain lung diseases. Today it is very little used, having been replaced by the manufacture of new antibiotics and other medicines.

The crude drug is collected only in the wild. It takes very many years for Iceland Moss to reach the size required by the drug market and this is also true of other lichens sometimes used in pharmaceutics, *Usnea* and *Cladonia* species for example. Central European countries import the drug mainly from Scandinavia and the Tyrol, but it is also collected in the Alps, the Giant Mountains and the Carpathians.

1. *Detail of the thallus*
   a) branching of the thallus
   b) cone-shaped lobe of thallus with fringed margin
2. *Whole lichen*

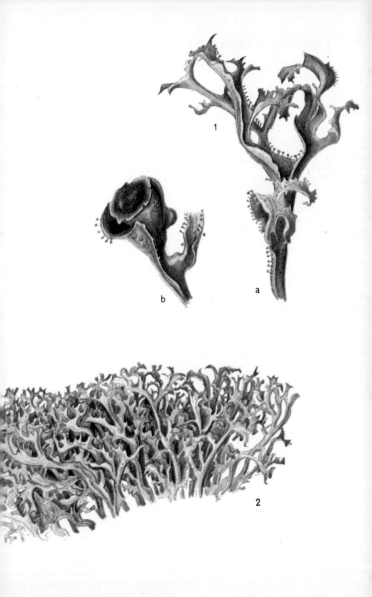

† *Chelidonium majus* L.

Greater Celandine

This is a perennial herb which flowers from May to September and grows in abundance in woods, at the roadside and on waste land, particularly on soils rich in nitrogen, from lowland to foothill elevations. It is found throughout the temperate — and in places also the arctic — regions of Eurasia. It has been introduced into North America in the area bordering the Atlantic.

The part generally collected for the crude drug are the top parts *(Herba chelidonii)*, gathered before the flowering stage from March until May. Rhizomes *(Radix chelidonii)* are gathered in autumn. To prevent undesirable changes in the drug it must be dried rapidly by artificial heat at temperatures not exceeding 60°C. The drug is odourless, and hot and bitter to the tongue. Because of the plant's toxicity great care must be taken in its collection. The drug contains up to 0.5 per cent of alkaloids, twelve of which have been isolated to date. In addition it contains organic acids to which the alkaloids are bound, namely malic acid, citric acid and chelidonic acid, traces of an unspecified essential oil and, in the fresh juice, other effective substances such as proteolytic enzymes. Also noteworthy are the anti-carcinogenic effects of certain chemical components, inapplicable as yet, however, because of their extreme toxicity.

The drug has a mild sedative action on the central nervous system; it relieves pain, relaxes spasms, raises the blood pressure, widens the coronary veins and stimulates the secretion of bile. It is used mainly in the form of specifics for the treatment of gall bladder disorders, including inflammation of the gall bladder, gallstones and hepatitis, but only under the supervision of a physician. Externally the fresh juice is used to remove warts.

The drug is gathered only in the wild.

1. *Part of the flowering plant*
2. *Fruits*
3. *Seed*

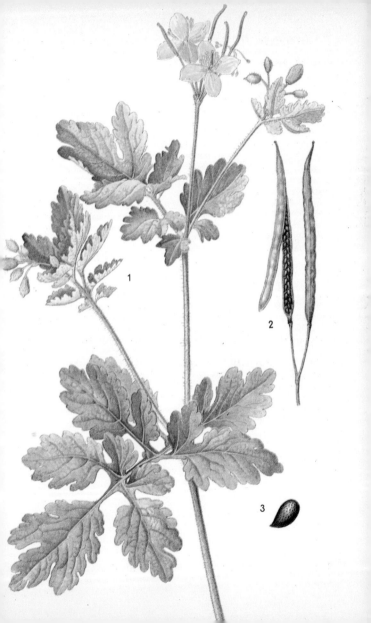

1

2

3

† *Claviceps purpurea* (FR.) TUL. Clavicipitaceae

Ergot Fungus

This is a spore-bearing fungus in which the dormant phase is a hard club-shaped body or sclerotium. The fungus is a parasitic growth which feeds on the ovaries of various grasses, mainly rye. Of practically cosmopolitan distribution it occurs in localities providing suitable host plants and conditions for its successful growth. It is found chiefly on grasses growing in the wild and practically no longer occurs on cultivated cereal grains as a result of the treatment given the seed prior to planting.

The crude drug is the purple sclerotium (Ergot), collected from ripening rye and dried in thin layers by natural heat. The drug is stored in cool, dry and well-ventilated storerooms. It must be protected against insect infestation. It is no longer used in its natural form but solely for the industrial isolation of alkaloids. Because of the great consumption of Ergot it is cultivated by the artificial 'infection' of rye grown only for this purpose, the infection and harvesting being mechanized. Ergot contains a number of toxic alkaloids. The basis of the alkaloids is lysergic acid from which further, therapeutically important substances are prepared. Ergot alkaloids affect smooth muscle and some of their derivatives have a pronounced action on the nervous system. Pharmaceutical preparations containing Ergot alkaloids or derivatives of lysergic acid may be prescribed only by a physician.

The drug is used in obstetrics to check uterine haemorrhage, block pain and eradicate inflammations of nervous origin, and in recent years also in psychiatry.

Today Ergot is a farm crop grown on rye in many countries of Europe, chiefly Czechoslovakia. Ergot was first cultivated artificially in Switzerland in about 1940.

1. *Sclerotia in infected rye*
2. *Sclerotia separated from host plant*
3. *Germinating sclerotium*

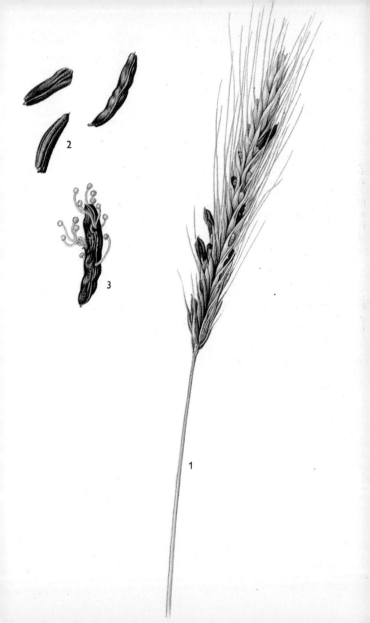

1
2
3

Cnicus benedictus L.

Compositae

Blessed Thistle

This annual herb flowers in June and July, and is indigenous to southern Europe and to south-west Asia. It was introduced into central Europe and has now become well established in the wild on sunny, stony slopes, at the roadside and on waste land. It is also found in many parts of the USSR, South Africa, the southern United States, Chile, Argentina and Uruguay.

The flowering top parts *(Herba cardui benedicti)* are collected for the drug market. These are cut before the inflorescence is fully opened and then dried in the shade. If artificial heat is used the temperature must not exceed 45° C. Collecting and further handling of the crude drug must be done with gloved hands because of the plant's thorniness. The crude drug is odourless and has a markedly bitter taste, owing to the presence of bitter principles, tannins, flavones, resins and traces of an essential oil and mucilage. It increases the flow of gastric secretions and has a mildly stimulating effect on bile secretion. In small doses it relieves digestive trouble but large doses should be avoided as they can cause gastric upsets. *Cnicus benedictus* is used with success as an extract in the treatment of gastric and digestive disorders. It forms a part of herbal tea mixtures and herbal alcoholic extracts and stomach bitters.

The drug is obtained mostly from cultivated plants. In mediaeval times this was a common medicinal herb of monastery gardens.

1. *Part of the flowering plant*
2. *Detail of inflorescence*

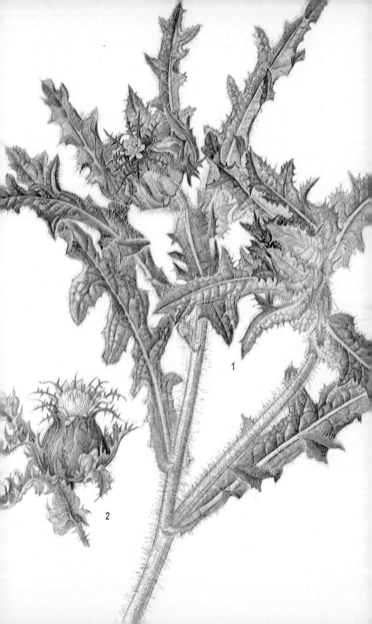

1

2

† *Colchicum autumnale* L.

Autumn Crocus

This perennial herb grows from a corm. It flowers from August to October and grows in great abundance in damp — usually mown, fertilized or regularly flooded — meadows and marshes, on road and railway banks and in alder groves, from lowland to foothill, sometimes also at alpine elevations. Its range of distribution includes western, southern, and parts of central and northern Europe. It is not found in the USSR, Greece and Turkey. It is cultivated in certain regions and is sometimes found wild in the area for a time.

The seeds *(Semen colchici)* and sometimes the corms *(Tuber colchici)* are collected for the drug market, the seeds in May and June, the corms in spring and autumn. The seeds must be ripe and must be dried further to prevent their becoming mouldy. Although formerly a common drug, the use of the corms for medicinal purposes is being abandoned because of the inconstant content of their active principles. All parts of the Autumn Crocus are extremely poisonous and great care must be taken in its collection. The active principles are alkaloids — chiefly colchicine — which effectively relieve pain in gout. Colchicine inhibits cell division (the so-called cytostatic effect); it is a strong cellular poison. Only preparations from pure alkaloids isolated from the seed are used, never the crude drug. Because of their high toxicity they are reliable medicines only when prescribed by a physician. They are used to relieve severe pain in gout, and experiments making use of their cytostatic action have been carried out in the treatment of cancer. In this case, of course, the high toxicity of colchicine is a serious drawback.

The drug is collected only in the wild.

1. *Non-flowering plant with corm and capsules*
2. *Flower*

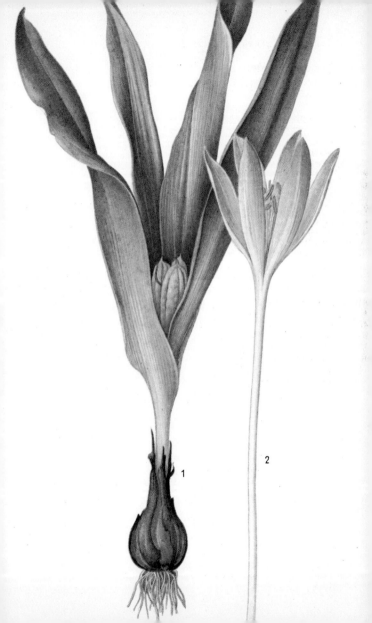

† *Convallaria majalis* L. Liliaceae

Lily-of-the-Valley

This perennial herb flowers in April and May, although frequently not at all in unsuitable localities. It grows abundantly, sometimes very thickly, in thin woodland — deciduous and mixed woods as well as coniferous forests — clearings and meadows, from lowland to subalpine elevations. The species is widespread in the temperate regions of the Northern Hemisphere; in North America it is found only in the Alleghenies. In Eurasia there are several species, *C. majalis* occurring only in Europe.

The flowering shoots *(Herba convallariae)* are collected for the drug market; they are cut at ground level at the beginning of the flowering season in May and June and dried without turning in thin layers in a shady and well-aired spot. If dried by artificial heat the temperature must not exceed 50° C. If properly dried the drug contains no brown flowers or leaves. It is odourless and has a sharp sweetish-bitter taste. When stored it should be protected from light and damp. Workers handling the drug may be subject to attacks of sneezing caused by saponins which irritate the mucous membrane. The drug contains toxic cardiac glycosides, as well as saponins. It affects cardiac activity and its action is similar to that of the glycosides of *Strophanthus*. The onset of the effect is rapid but so is its termination. The drug also has a favourable diuretic action so that no concentration of glycosides in the body has been observed. Medicines made from Lily-of-the-Valley should be prescribed only by a physician. They are used in the treatment of cardiac insufficiency either in the form of a tincture or as a specific.

The drug is collected only in the wild. It is not cultivated for pharmaceutical purposes.

1. *Flowering plant*
2. *Fruits*

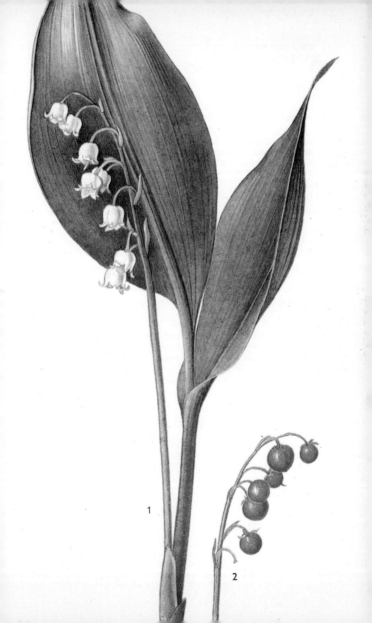

1

2

Coriandrum sativum L.

Umbelliferae

Coriander

An annual herb flowering in June and July, Coriander is probably indigenous only to the eastern Mediterranean countries where today it is a common field weed. It is practically worldwide in cultivation and is often found as a temporary escape in fields and vineyards, near warehouses and railway stations and on waste land, from lowland to foothill elevations in warmer climates — the Mediterranean, central Europe, eastern Asia, and parts of North and South America.

The fruits *(Fructus coriandri)* are collected for medicinal purposes. These are obtained from the cultivated plant by threshing in the same way as the fruits of Anise, Fennel and Caraway. When crushed the drug has a penetratingly pungent odour and taste. It contains 0.4—1 per cent of an essential oil. It stimulates the flow of digestive secretions, is useful as a carminative and in the treatment of intestinal disorders, and has antispasmodic and expectorant properties.

It is used internally in the form of an infusion, primarily in relieving flatulence and stomach cramps and in stimulating the appetite. Externally, it is used in ointments for the treatment of rheumatism and arthritis. Coriander, however, is used far more frequently as a culinary herb and flavouring agent in meat dishes, sauces and the fish-tinning industry. Oil distilled from the seeds, besides being used in the food industry, pharmaceutics and perfumery, also serves as a raw material for the production of aromatic substances such as linalool, citral and ionone. The volatile oil distilled from the aerial parts has a rather disagreeable odour as does the entire fresh plant.

Coriander is cultivated in many countries of Europe and Asia, but chiefly in the USSR.

1. *Inflorescence*
2. *Fruits*
3. *Detail of fruit*

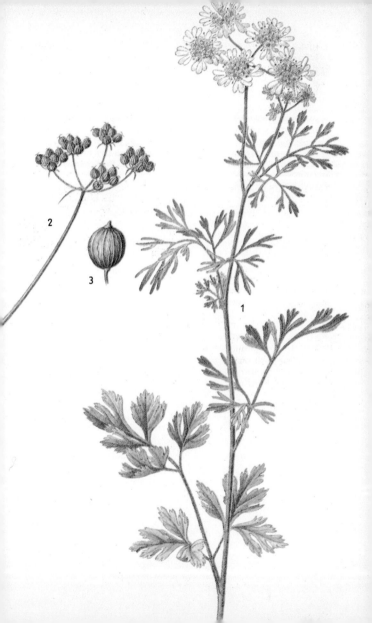

Crataegus oxyacantha L. Rosaceae

Hawthorn

Hawthorn is a shrub or small tree, which flowers in May and June, commonly in scrub, thin woodland and hedges from lowland to foothill elevations, and very occasionally at mountain elevations. It is distributed throughout central Europe from the Pyrenees, central England, southern Sweden east to the Baltic countries and the western shores of the Black Sea; in the south it is also found in Sicily and Greece. It is sometimes cultivated.

The flowers *(Flos crataegi)* and fruits *(Fructus crataegi)* are collected for medicinal purposes, the former being picked before they are at their best in May and June, the ripe fruits in September and October. Both are dried in the shade at temperatures below 40° C (flowers) and 50° C (fruits). Badly dried flowers turn brown. The crude drug from the flowers, which is thought to be the more effective, has an unpleasant smell. The fruits are odourless and have a faintly bitter taste. The most important active principles are the flavonoids, and a mixture of triterpenic acids. They act as vasodilators and cardiants and reduce blood pressure.

The drug is employed internally in the form of an infusion or as part of ready-made pharmaceutical preparations. Frequently fresh flowers and berries are used instead of the crude drug. They are effective in the treatment of cardiac disorders of nervous origin, insomnia, hypertension and menopausal upsets. They exert a beneficial action in incipient arteriosclerosis, and in the period of convalescence following a stroke.

The drug is collected only in the wild. The flowers of *Crataegus monogyna* JACQ., which grows in similar localities in Europe, from western Siberia to the Himalayas and in North Africa, are also collected. Drugs sold on the market are usually a mixture of the two species.

1. *Flowers*
2. *Fruits*

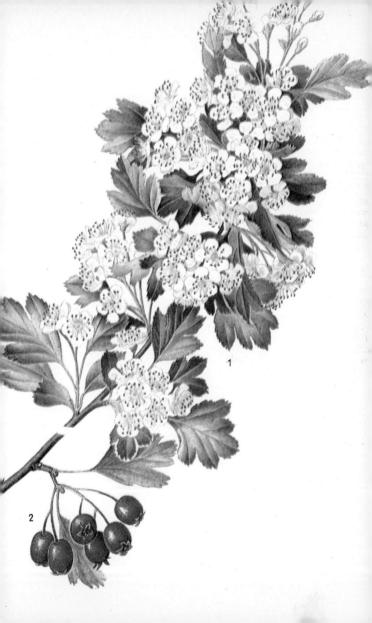

1

2

Crocus sativus L.

Saffron

This is a perennial herb with a flattened underground corm, which flowers from September to November. Although a much-cultivated plant, its native home is the eastern Mediterranean region extending to the Middle East.

The stigmas *(Stigmata croci)*, which are plucked out of the open flowers, are collected for the drug market. They are dried first in the shade and then on fine mesh over a small fire. Collecting is laborious, up to 200,000 stigmas being required to yield 1 kilogram of the drug. The drug is a bright reddish-orange and has a pungent odour and taste. It must be stored in tightly stoppered tins because it easily loses its colour, aroma and flavour. As Saffron is such a costly drug, it is often mixed with raw materials of a similar colour, such as the flowers of Marigold or Safflower. It contains mainly pigments and a minute quantity of essential oil. It allays pain and acts as an antispasmodic.

It was once used as a home remedy but is no longer employed in medical practice. However, it is much used to season and colour foods, especially oriental dishes. Excessive quantities of Saffron may cause serious poisoning by local irritation of the mucous membranes followed by spasmodic contractions and bleeding.

Today the drug is only of marginal importance partly because of its expense and the enormous quantities of flowers necessary to yield only a tiny amount of the drug. It is grown mostly in Spain, where the yearly production is about 100,000 kilograms. In mediaeval times the cultivation of Saffron was widespread throughout the whole Mediterranean region and central Europe, where it was used as a dye. In England it used to be cultivated at Saffron Walden and even now can be found growing wild in that area. It is also grown in southern France, Italy, Sicily, Hungary, Greece, Turkey, Iran, India and China.

1. *Flowering plant*
2. *Detail of stigma*

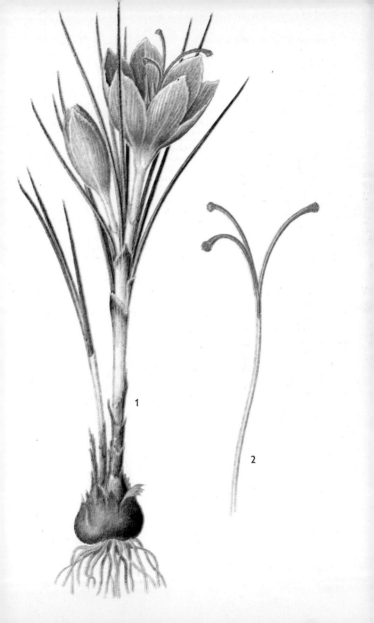

Cuminum cyminum L.

Cumin

An annual herb flowering in June and July, Cumin is probably indigenous to the eastern Mediterranean countries, but according to more recent knowledge, it is also native in Turkestan alongside the Amu Darya and Syr Darya rivers in the Kizil-kum desert region. The cultivation of this plant was introduced to Egypt, south-eastern and southern Europe in ancient times.

The parts used for the drug are the fruits *(Fructus cumini)*, which are collected when ripe in August and September, then dried and cleaned after threshing. The drug is very aromatic, containing 2.5—5 per cent of an essential oil. It contains tannins and oil, in addition to the essential oil. It acts as a carminative, stimulates the flow of digestive secretions and also lactation.

Nowadays, the drug is only rarely used; it is taken internally in the form of an infusion or as a component of herbal tea mixtures in the same way as Caraway. It has proved effective in the treatment of dyspepsia, colic and flatulence. The volatile oil distilled from the fruits is used in perfumery. The seeds are used as a seasoning by the food industry in the making of cheese — especially in the Netherlands — in bread and rolls as a substitute for Caraway, and in certain liqueurs.

Cumin has been grown for centuries in the Mediterranean region, chiefly in Egypt, Morocco, Malta and Syria. It is also cultivated in India, China, Ethiopia and recently in North and South America — especially Chile. It was previously grown in central Europe, also, where to this day it sometimes finds its way in among shipments of grain and seed, establishing a foothold and growing wild for a time.

1. *Umbels with fruits*
2. *Detail of fruit*
3. *Inflorescence*

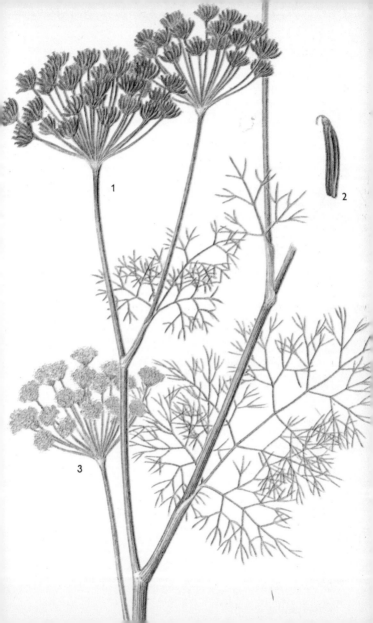

† *Datura stramonium* L. Solanaceae

Thorn Apple, Jimson Weed

This annual herb, flowering from June to October, is most probably native to the north-eastern regions of North America from whence it was introduced to other parts of America, Europe and the rest of the world. It has a scattered, sometimes locally abundant, distribution on waste ground, at roadsides and near human habitations from lowland to foothill elevations in most of the temperate and subtropical parts of the Northern Hemisphere. Today it can be found in waste places such as city dumps in practically any country in the world.

Most of the crude drug is in the leaves *(Folium stramonii)* of flowering plants, only rarely in the ripe seeds *(Semen stramonii)*. The leaves are dried in the shade or by artificial heat at temperatures not exceeding 50° C. The drug has an overpowering smell and a bitter-salty flavour. As the plant is extremely poisonous great care must be taken in its collection, the collector wearing gloves and some form of protection for the eyes and mouth. The leaves contain toxic tropane alkaloids in quantities of up to 0.5 per cent, in addition the seeds contain up to 20 per cent of fixed oil. The action of the tropane alkaloids, and their uses, are the same as those of Henbane and Belladonna.

The drug is sometimes used in anti-asthmatic cigarettes, otherwise practically not at all, pure alkaloids in doses prescribed by a physician being employed instead.

Jimson Weed is generally gathered wild. When it is cultivated for medicinal purposes, as a rule those species that are rich in scopolamine are grown, such as *Datura innoxia* P. MILL. (tropical regions of America) and *D. metel* L. (tropical and subtropical regions of Asia and Africa) or cultivars of *D. stramonium* L., principally those with spineless capsules and a higher alkaloid content. The plant has been known in Spain since the second half of the sixteenth century from where it spread to other countries as a garden ornamental. A century later garden escapes had already become established in the wild.

1. *Part of the plant with flower and fruit*
2. *Seed*

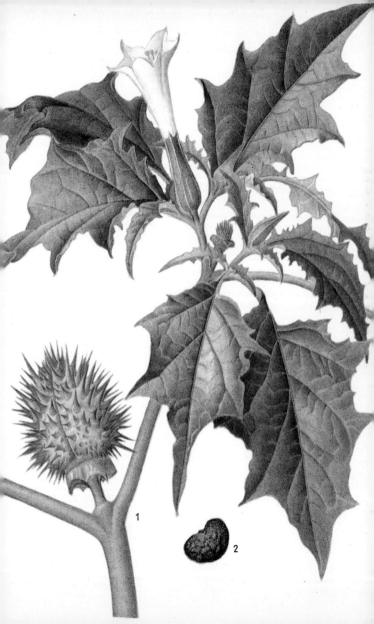

1

2

† *Digitalis lanata* EHRH. Scrophulariaceae

This is a biennial or perennial herb, flowering from June to August, which grows in thickets, light woodland and forest clearings from hilly country to mountain elevations. The range of distribution extends from the mountains of northern Hungary to the mountains of the Middle East.

The drug is obtained from the leaves *(Folium digitalis lanatae)*, which are cut just above the ground from the first year's growth in dry, sunny weather in October. Because it is cultivated as a crop plant for medicinal purposes it is dried by artificial heat, which must not exceed 50° C, in well-ventilated drying rooms. It must be stored in dry conditions. The drug, which has a disagreeable, bitter flavour, contains highly potent cardiac glycosides (lanatosides) and saponins. The lanatoside content depends on many external and internal factors.

The glycosides of this drug are the most potent cardiac medicine known. One drawback, however, is that in prolonged application there is a tendency for the glycosides to build up to a dangerous level. The drug is administered only when and as prescribed by a physician, in the form of precisely dosed preparations such as tablets, drops or injections. It is used in the treatment of heart disease, and the regulation of heart rate, rhythm, tone, contraction and conduction of impulses.

D. lanata is cultivated commercially in Switzerland, Austria, Germany, Hungary and Czechoslovakia and has largely replaced the use of Foxglove *(Digitalis purpurea* L.*)* on the continent because of its greater potency.

1. *Part of the stem with leaves*
2. *Part of the stem with flowers*
   Both 1. and 2. are from a plant in its second year.

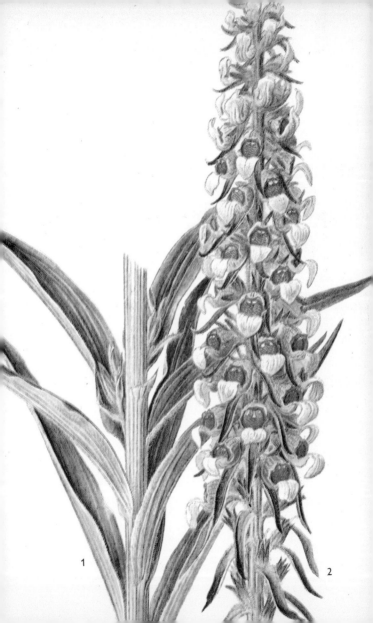

1

2

Drosera rotundifolia L.

Droseraceae

Sundew

This is a perennial, insectivorous herb, which flowers from June to August and has a scattered distribution on wet moors and peat bogs, and sometimes on the fringes of small ponds, usually on lime-free substrates from lowland to mountain elevations. The distribution includes the arctic and temperate regions of the Northern Hemisphere and it is believed to be indigenous to North America.

The leaves and flowers *(Herba droserae rotundifoliae)* are collected for medicinal purposes at the beginning of the flowering stage from June to August. They are pinched off at ground level and spread out to dry in thin layers in a shady and well-ventilated spot. They are never dried by artificial heat. The drug is odourless, bitter and stringent to the tongue. The active principles which bring about the therapeutic effects have not been precisely determined to date but it is believed that they are caused by the whole complex of constituents. The drug exerts a diuretic action, lowers the blood sugar level and relieves congestion of the respiratory passages.

It is used internally as an infusion or tincture and as a component of herbal tea mixtures in stubborn coughs, asthma and bronchitis. It is popular as a home remedy for diseases associated with middle and old age, chiefly arteriosclerosis and hypertension. More detailed investigation of the drug is prevented by its limited availability and also because in many places it is a protected plant.

The herb is gathered only in the wild, its collection being extremely difficult and tedious. The aerial parts of other species, such as *D. angelica* HUDS. (from the same regions as *D. rotundifolia* L.), and the South African *D. capensis* L., are also sold for medicinal purposes; they are believed to be less effective but there are no grounds to support this opinion.

Flowering plant. Prominent glandular leaves arranged in a ground rosette.

122

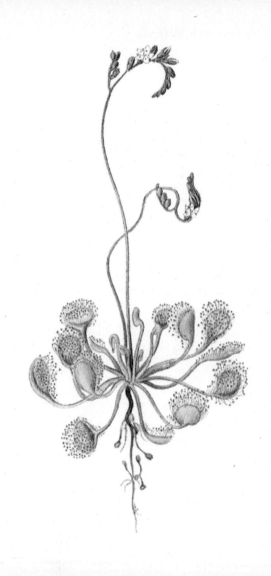

Euphrasia officinalis L.

Scrophulariaceae

Eyebright

This is an annual, very variable herb, which flowers from May to October; it is indigenous to central Europe, and plentiful in fields and meadows.

The flowering aerial parts *(Herba euphrasiae)* are collected for medicinal purposes. These are gathered mostly in summer and autumn and are either dried in thin layers in the shade or by artificial heat at temperatures not exceeding 40° C. If properly dried the leaves and flowers should not change colour during the process. The drug has a bitter taste and is odourless. The active principles are not precisely known. They are believed to be tannins, resins with disinfectant properties, and possibly glycosides. In any case the drug acts as an astringent and reduces inflammation.

It is used externally, as a rule, in compresses, or as an extract in douches and eye lotions, or internally as a tea in digestive or gall bladder disorders.

The drug — generally consisting of several independent species of *Euphrasia* — is collected only in the wild.

Flowering plant

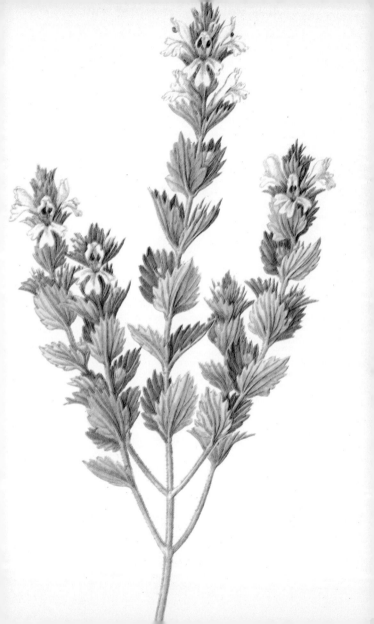

Foeniculum vulgare P. MILL.   Umbelliferae

Fennel

Fennel is a biennial or perennial plant, flowering from July to October, believed to be indigenous only in the area extending from the eastern Mediterranean to Iran. It is found wild — often established or introduced — in western and central Europe, China, Japan, Ethiopia, South Africa, North and South America and New Zealand. It grows on city dumps, bare ground, vineyards, and alongside roads and railways in warmer climates.

The parts collected are the fruits *(Fructus foeniculi)*. The plants are harvested before complete maturation of the fruit, tied into bunches and left to ripen fully. Then they are taken on large canvas sheets to be threshed. After cleaning, the fruits are further dried. The drug has a pleasant, spicy odour and a burning, sweet taste. It contains 2.5—6 per cent of an essential oil. It exerts a disinfectant and anti-inflammatory action, primarily on the respiratory and digestive organs, and has an antispasmodic effect on smooth muscle. It is said to stimulate lactation. In excessively high doses, however, it causes spasmodic contractions and delusions.

It is used, in the form of an infusion or in herbal teas and syrups, as an expectorant in the treatment of diseases of the upper respiratory tract and as an anodyne and disinfectant in gastric and intestinal catarrh accompanied by flatulence and spasms. The volatile oil recovered from the seeds is used not only in pharmaceutics but also in the food industry. The fruits are a condiment.

The drug is obtained only from cultivated plants. The chief suppliers are Germany, France, Bulgaria, Hungary and the USSR.

1. *Top part with flowering and seed umbels*
2. *Detail of fruit*
3. *Detail of flower*

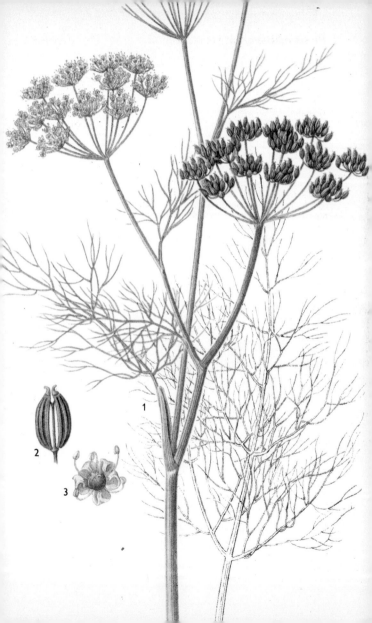

1

2

3

Frangula alnus P. MILL.   Rhamnaceae

Alder Buckthorn, Black Dogwood

This shrub flowers in May and June and grows fairly abundantly in damp deciduous and coniferous woods, coastal thickets, alongside forest streams, on screes and generally near water from lowland to mountain elevations. It is distributed throughout most of Europe and occurs in Siberia, south-west and central Asia and perhaps also North Africa. Cultivation has resulted in its propagation in the wild in North America. Its range of distribution in central Asia and North Africa has not been precisely delimited as yet.

The part used for extraction of the active principles is the bark *(Cortex frangulae)*, peeled in April and May from young, severed branches. It is dried in the sun or at a temperature not exceeding 45° C. For medicinal purposes the drug is used only after it has been kept for a year because when fresh it causes nausea, retching and cramps, provoked by the anthrone glycosides. The drug is odourless and has a sweetish, faintly bitter taste. It contains anthraquinone glycosides, tannins, bitter principles and other constituents. Their action is cathartic and stimulates bile secretion.

The drug is used internally as a powder, in herbal tea mixtures, in macerated form, as an extract and with a mixture of glycosides in various preparations to relieve constipation.

The drug is collected only in the wild. In view of the demand, however, the establishment of plantations is being considered. The chief suppliers are Poland, Czechoslovakia, Yugoslavia and the USSR. The first authentic records of its medicinal use are from the early fourteenth century.

1. *Flowering branch*
2. *Detail of flower*
3. *Fruit*
4. *Bark*

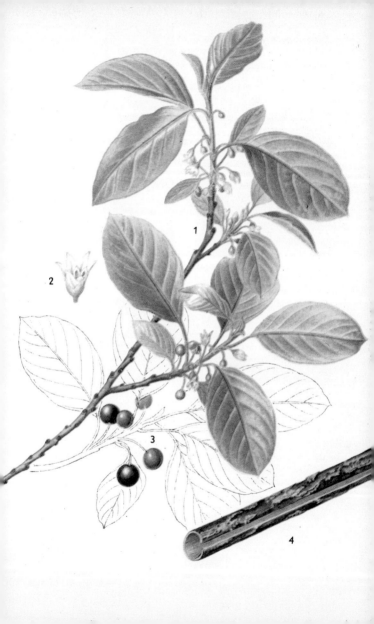

1   2   3   4

Gentiana lutea L. Gentianaceae

Gentian

This perennial herb, flowering from June to August, grows in masses on pastures, meadows, screes and rocky slopes and amidst thickets at high altitudes, mostly on limey substrates. It occurs in the mountainous areas of southern and central Europe and western Turkey. In some parts of the regions where it is indigenous it has been wiped out by collecting for the drug market and by transplantation to gardens.

The drug is found chiefly in the rhizomes and roots *(Radix gentianae)* collected in September and October. These are washed and dried rapidly at temperatures not exceeding 50°C. The dried drug is yellow-brown (pale yellow inside), has a distinct and pleasant odour, and a sweetish, later strong, markedly bitter taste. It contains bitter principles (about 2 per cent) and also small amounts of tannins, mucilages and sugars. The bitter principles increase the flow of digestive secretions and stimulate the appetite.

Internally the drug is used in the form of infusions, tinctures and extracts as a tonic and stomachic, in eradicating intestinal worms, and in veterinary medicine. It is employed by the food industry in the preparation of bitter beverages and aperitifs in which case use is made of the fermented drug. Fermentation takes place when the roots have been gathered and piled in heaps before being dried. The fermented roots are brownish-red in colour and are far more aromatic and less bitter than the unfermented roots.

The drug is generally collected in the wild but because these plants are rapidly disappearing it is beginning to be cultivated. The market drug often consists of other species as well as the one listed here.

1. *Rhizome*
2. *Flower stem*

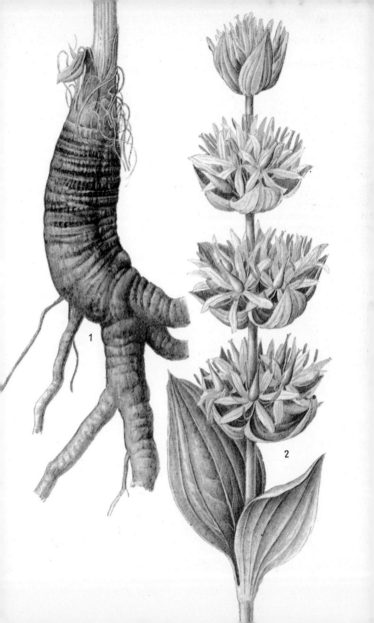

Herniaria glabra L. Caryophyllaceae

Glabrous Rupture-wort

This is an annual to perennial herb flowering from July to September. It has a very local distribution on paths, sandy fields, pastures, alongside byways, and between the stones of pavements and river dams, from lowland to foothill elevations. It is almost completely restricted to quartzy substrates. The range of distribution embraces the temperate regions of Europe, western Asia and the Mediterranean.

The aerial parts *(Herba herniariae)* are collected during the flowering period from July to September and left to dry in a well-ventilated spot or else dried in drying rooms by artificial heat at temperatures not exceeding 45° C. The drug is faintly aromatic and causes a scratchy sensation on the tongue. It contains saponins that act as haemolytics, coumarins, flavones and traces of an essential oil. It has a diuretic effect and an antispasmodic action on the urinary organs.

It is used internally in the form of an infusion, in herbal tea mixtures and as an extract to treat chronic inflammation of the urinary bladder, kidney stones and inflammation of the prostate gland.

The drug is collected only in the wild. Attempts at cultivation with the exception of semi-cultures on the banks of waterways, have been unsuccessful to date.

H. hirsuta L., which grows in localities similar to the above species, is also gathered. The range of distribution embraces western, central and southern Europe, central Asia, the Punjab and Ethiopia.

Flowering plant

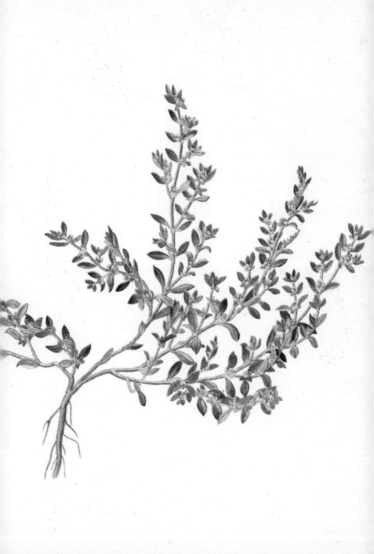

Humulus lupulus L.   Cannabinaceae

Common Hop

The Hop is a perennial, climbing herb with stems twining in a clockwise direction. It flowers from June to September. It is most probably indigenous only to southern Europe, south-west Asia and North America; today it is widely scattered in the temperate regions of the Northern Hemisphere. Hops grow fairly freely in damp coastal thickets and in alder groves from lowland to hilly country. They are occasionally found in foothills and at higher elevations.

The parts collected for the drug are the pistillate catkins called strobiles *(Strobuli lupuli)* or — now only in small measure — the grains on the surface of the bracts that form the strobiles *(Glandulae lupuli* — lupulin*)*. The strobiles are collected before maturation in late August and early September and dried at temperatures not exceeding 40° C. The grains, if these are desired, are knocked out of the dried strobiles. Both drugs have an aromatic odour and characteristic bitter flavour, though aging causes a loss of aroma and efficiency. The drug must therefore not be more than a year old and must be stored in closed containers in a dry, dark place. Both drugs contain bitter principles as well as a small amount of an essential oil. Their most pronounced therapeutic effect is their sedative action. They check the multiplication of numerous bacteria and have a mild diuretic action. Hormonal effects have also been demonstrated.

Both drugs are used only to a limited extent today in the form of an infusion or extract or as a component of specifics for insomnia, as a mild diuretic in prostate afflictions and as a digestant. The Hop is no longer important as a drug, its principal use being in the brewing of beer. The volatile oil recovered from Hop is used in small quantities in perfumery (cologne), and its composition varies according to the geographic origin of the plant.

Hops are cultivated principally in Europe, the United States, Chile and Australia.

1. *Part of plant with pistillate catkins*
2. *Detail of male flower*
3. *Detail of female flower*

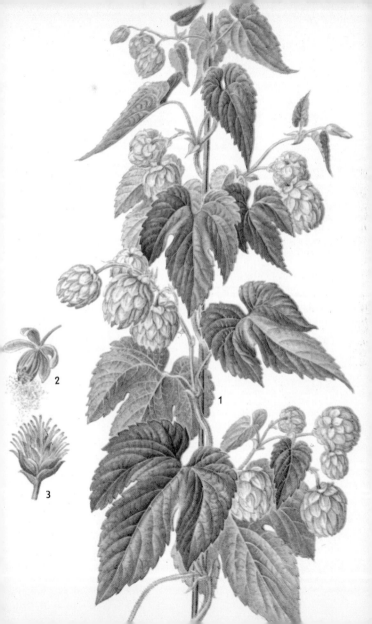

† *Hyoscyamus niger* L.

Solanaceae

Henbane

Henbane is generally a biennial — less frequently an annual — herb, flowering from June to October and growing on waste ground, on fallow land, and by the roadside from lowland to foothill elevations. It is most probably indigenous only to the Mediterranean countries. The range of distribution embraces practically the whole of Eurasia, excepting the northernmost regions, and North Africa. The plant has been introduced into eastern Asia, North America and Australia.

The parts serving for extraction of the active principles are the leaves *(Folium hyoscyami)* and sometimes also the seeds *(Semen hyoscyami)*. The leaves of flowering plants are gathered in July and August and dried carefully by natural or artifical heat. The drug has a peculiar foetid odour and a sharp, bitter-salty taste. The seeds are gathered before they are ripe. The top parts with the fruit are cut off, left to dry in a well-ventilated place, then threshed and cleaned. The plant is extremely poisonous and therefore should never be gathered except by a qualified collector who knows how to take the proper precautions. The drug from the leaves contains toxic tropane alkaloids and tannins. Tropane alkaloids irritate and may even have a paralytic effect on the central nervous system, they inhibit the flow of saliva and widen the pupil of the eye. Modern medicinal therapy employs the leaves only as a component in anti-asthmatic preparations or in medicines relieving spasms of smooth muscle.

Because tropane alkaloids are recovered principally from Deadly Nightshade *(Atropa belladonna)* or Jimson Weed *(Datura stramonium)* neither collection nor cultivation of this plant are of any importance. Occasionally there is a demand for the drug from other species of Henbane, such as *H. muticus* L. Henbane has been known as a medicinal plant since ancient times. It is often found in waste places such as city dumps.

1. *Top part of a flowering plant*
2. *Calyx containing fruit*
3. *Fruit*
4. *Seed*

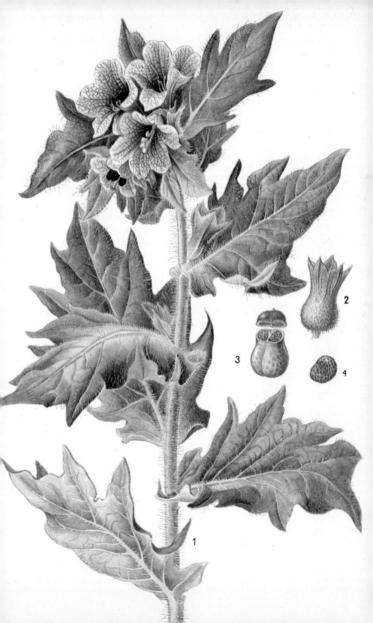

Hypericum perforatum L. Hypericaceae

St John's Wort

This is a perennial herb, flowering from May to September which has a wide distribution in open woods, forest clearings, grassland, hedgerows and at roadsides and on waste land, from lowland to subalpine elevations. It is distributed throughout the temperate regions of Europe and western Asia, in North Africa and the Canary Islands. It has become naturalized in eastern Asia, North and South America, Australia and New Zealand.

The drug is concentrated principally in the top of the flower and stem *(Herba hyperici)*, which are gathered at the beginning of the flowering period. The lower parts of the stems are not collected nor flower heads past their prime because the drug must not contain any seeds. The flowers are dried — in layers or tied in bunches — as rapidly as possible in a well-ventilated spot or by artificial heat at temperatures not exceeding 40° C. The drug has a faint scent and slightly bitter taste. It contains colouring matter, glycosides and vitamins, about 10 per cent of tannins and 0.1 per cent of an essential oil.

It has a favourable action on the basic metabolism and secretion of bile, and improves blood circulation; it also has anti-inflammatory and healing properties. It is used internally as an infusion or as a specific in gastric and intestinal catarrh accompanied by diarrhoea, to stimulate the appetite, and in the treatment of depression and disturbed sleep. Externally, it is generally applied in macerated oil form to wounds, hemorrhoids and burns.

The drug is collected only in the wild, but in view of the rising demand attempts are being made to cultivate it.

Flowering top

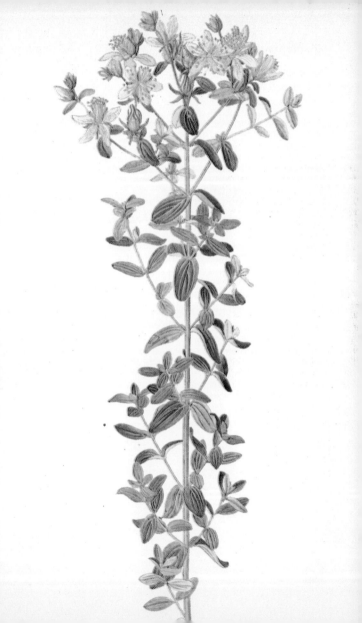

Hyssopus officinalis L.

Labiatae

Hyssop

A semi-shrub flowering from June to August, Hyssop grows on dry, rocky slopes in full sun, especially on limestone hills and on south-facing mountain slopes, from Spain to the Caspian Sea and northern Iran. In view of its long history of cultivation it is difficult to determine the boundaries of the species' original distribution. For example, in Algeria it grows only in the wild, but as a naturalized wild plant. It was introduced into North America.

The flowering shoots *(Herba hyssopi)* are collected for the drug market from July to August. They are dried in the shade in thin layers or strung up in bunches to dry at normal temperatures. In drying rooms they are dried by artificial heat at temperatures not exceeding 40° C. The drug has a spicy scent and slightly bitter taste. It contains 0.2—1 per cent of an essential oil, about 8 per cent of tannins, a flavonoid glycoside, and probably other substances. Its action is the same as that of Sage. It inhibits the secretion of the sweat glands and alleviates cough and hoarseness. The tannins have an astringent effect.

The drug is used internally, chiefly in home remedies as an infusion, to limit sweating, ease coughs, relax spasms in digestive upsets and to aid digestion. Externally, it is used as a gargle. The drug yields a volatile oil used for the same purposes. In larger doses it causes cramps. Fresh as well as dried leaves are used as a flavouring in soups, sauces, and roast meats, the volatile oil is used as a component of seasoning essences — in combination with Marjoram and Tarragon oils — and also with the essential oils of certain species of Wormwood *(Artemisia)* in flavouring the liqueur absinthe in Switzerland and southern France.

The herb is collected wild in the Mediterranean and central Asia, and is also cultivated in Germany, France, the USSR and India.

1. *Flowering plant*
2. *Detail of a flower*

140

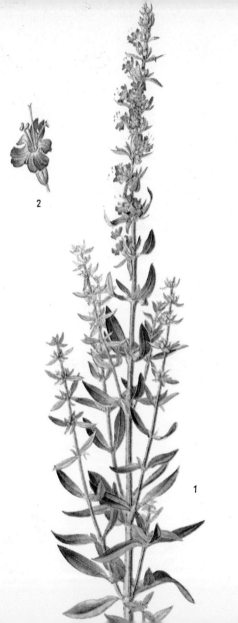

1

2

Inula helenium L.

Compositae

Elecampane

This is a perennial herb flowering from June to October, which is most probably indigenous only to central Asia, although some authorities believe it to be native to the Appenines and the Balkans. It grows wild in many parts of Europe, and in Asia Minor, Japan and North America as self-sown seedlings from cultivated plants; it has also become naturalized in places difficult of access.

The rhizomes and roots *(Radix helenii)* of cultivated second-year plants are collected for medicinal purposes from September to October. They are washed quickly, the larger roots being cut in half, and then dried by artificial heat at temperatures not exceeding 45° C. Because the drug is very hygroscopic it must be stored in tightly closed containers. It has a pungent odour and bitter flavour. It contains 1—3 per cent of an essential oil which is solid at normal temperatures —the so-called camphor 'helenin'. Besides the essential oil there are also small quantities of bitter principles and other substances which have not yet been fully investigated. The essential oil stimulates the flow of digestive secretions and has a mildly diuretic action; it also acts as a vermicide.

The drug is used internally as an infusion, as a component in herbal tea mixtures and in specifics to diminish the cough reflex, in gastric insufficiency and intestinal catarrh, and as a subsidiary medicine in diabetes. It is employed as a vermicide in combination with santonin. It is also a component of herbal tea mixtures used in gall bladder treatment. Externally, it is applied to recalcitrant wounds and as a mouthwash for inflamed gums. The distilled volatile oil is used not only in medicine but also in perfumery.

The chief sources of supply are plants cultivated in the Netherlands, Belgium, France, Germany, Yugoslavia, Poland, Hungary and North America. In Roman times the rhizome was served as a vegetable as well as being used for medicinal purposes.

1. *Aerial part with inflorescences*
2. *Rhizome*

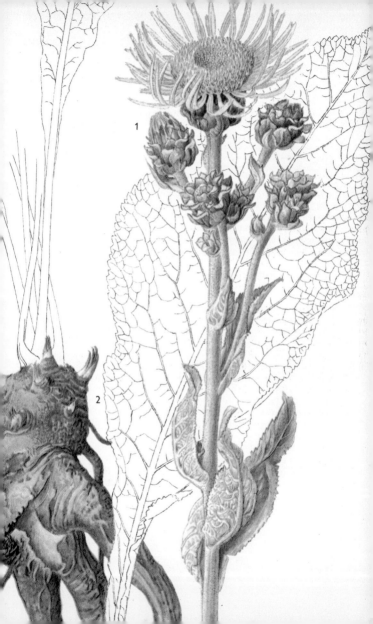

Juniperus communis L.

Cupressaceae

Common Juniper

This is a shrub of varying habit, sometimes a small tree, which flowers in April and May and has a fairly common but rather local distribution on chalk downs, heaths and moors and as undergrowth in open pine and birchwoods from lowland to mountain elevations. At high altitudes it occurs as a prostrate shrub — ssp. *nana* (WILLD.) BRIQ. It is distributed throughout the arctic and temperate regions of the Northern Hemisphere, but is absent from all but the northernmost parts of China.

The fruits or berries are used for the extraction of the active principles *(Fructus juniperi)* and very occasionally the wood *(Lignum juniperi)*, also. The ripe fruits are collected in September and October by shaking the tree over large canvas sheets. After cleaning, the berries are dried in thin layers in a shaded, well-ventilated spot. They have a resinous odour and sweetish taste and contain up to 2 per cent of an essential oil, the composition of which differs according to the origin of the drug. It also contains tannins, flavonoid glycosides, resins and about 30 per cent of invert sugar. The drug and essential oil have both diuretic and disinfectant properties.

The berries are used internally as an infusion and component of herbal teas in the treatment of inflammation of the urinary passages; they should not, however, be taken in serious kidney disorders or pregnancy. In the case of digestive upsets the drug is used for its stimulating effect on the flow of gastric secretions. Externally it is used in anti-rheumatic alcoholic ointments and baths. It is frequently used in veterinary medicine. A volatile oil is isolated from the berries commercially, being used especially in gin and liqueurs. The berries are also used as a condiment and the wood in curing smoked meat.

The drug is collected only in the wild.

1. *Flowering branch*
2. *Fruit-bearing branch*

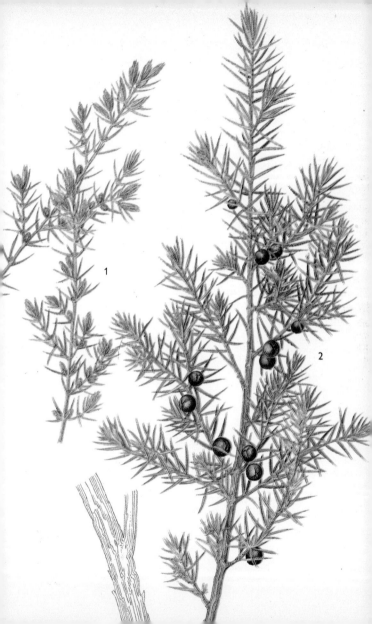

1

2

Linum usitatissimum L.

Linaceae

Flax

Flax is an annual herb of cultivated origin which flowers from June to August. The type plant is considered to be the Mediterranean perennial or biennial Narrow-leaved Flax, *L. angustifolium* HUDS. The oldest region of Flax cultivation is the Middle East. Today Flax is cultivated for the oil extracted from its seeds (large-seeded cultivars), for its fibres (small-seeded cultivars), and as combined oil-fibre cultivars practically throughout the world, excepting the tropics and coldest regions.

The seeds *(Semen lini)* are collected for medicinal purposes as soon as they are ripe. After threshing and cleaning the seeds are left to dry. The drug is odourless, mucilaginous when crushed and has a bland, oily taste. It contains up to 6 per cent of mucilage, and 30—40 per cent of fixed oil and protein substances. It has a mild laxative effect, soothes pain and exerts an anti-inflammatory action. In medicine it is placed together with other oils of similar composition in the class of vitamin-like substances which have a beneficial effect on skin rashes, burns, psoriasis and other skin diseases.

The drug is used internally in strained macerated form (in cold water) as a mild laxative and subsidiary medicine in inflammations of the respiratory, intestinal and urinary tracts. Externally, crushed seeds mixed with water are used to make hot poultices for the treatment of purulent and inflammatory skin disorders. The drug is obtained chiefly from cultivars especially bred for their higher oil content. Linseed oil is of great importance in the manufacture of paints and varnishes but the principal use of the plant is in the manufacture of thread and cloth from the fibres.

The chief growers of Flax are the USSR, India and the United States. Cultivation of the plant was known in Mesopotamia and Egypt as early as 5,000 BC.

Flowering plant

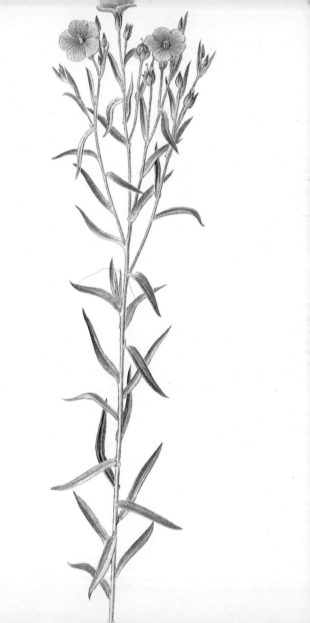

Majorana hortensis MOENCH
(Origanum majorana L.*)*

Labiatae

Marjoram

This is an annual to biennial herbaceous plant, flowering from July to September, which is indigenous to the area extending from Libya and Egypt through Arabia to India. Sometimes south-west Africa only is given as the place of origin. In the Mediterranean region, where it has been cultivated since ancient times, it has become naturalized as a perennial herbaceous plant to semi-shrub. It is also found growing in the wild in some parts of central Europe but does not become permanently established there.

The active principles are found chiefly in the aerial parts *(Herba majoranae)*, which are gathered before the flowering period, generally in June and July. They are dried in thin layers in a well-ventilated place or in drying rooms at a temperature not exceeding 40° C. The drug has an agreeable spicy smell and taste and is stored in tightly covered containers. It contains up to 2 per cent of an essential oil. The composition of the essential oil is fairly constant even in drugs of different origin. Besides the oil bitter substances and mucilages are also present. The active principles in the drug aid digestion, relieve flatulence, act as an intestinal antispasmodic and stimulate the secretion of bile.

The drug is used internally as an infusion in digestive upsets, flatulence, intestinal colic and diarrhoea. It should not be taken during pregnancy. Externally, it is used as a bath additive for the treatment of recalcitrant wounds. Marjoram is a popular flavouring but must be used only in small amounts for larger quantities have a stupefying effect. It is used to flavour meat dishes, and in making salamis and other sorts of sausage. The drug generally sold on the market is German Marjoram which contains the leaves, flowering shoots and part of the stems, while French Marjoram consists only of stripped leaves and the flower heads.

Marjoram has been cultivated in the Mediterranean countries for centuries and is still widely cultivated today, chiefly in Germany, Hungary and Czechoslovakia, as well as parts of Asia and in North America.

1. *Flowering plant*
2. *Detail of flower*

148

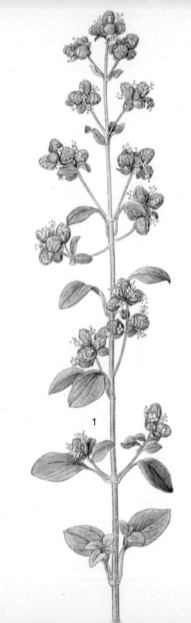

1

2

Malva silvestris Malvaceae
subsp. **mauritiana** (L.) A. *et* GR.

Mallow

This is a biennial to perennial herb, flowering from May to October, which is indigenous from the southern Mediterranean region to sub-tropical Asia. It is grown chiefly in central Europe as an ornamental plant, principally in outdoor gardens, and in some places grows wild. It rarely occurs as an introduced plant which has become temporarily established.

The parts collected for medicinal purposes are the leaves *(Folium malvae mauritianae)* and flowers *(Flos malvae mauritianae)*. They are gathered in dry weather during the flowering period, from June to September, and are dried rapidly by artificial heat at a temperature not exceeding 40° C. The dried flowers are dark blue. Leaves attacked by rust — a common trouble with plants of this family — must be removed. The drug is odourless and has a bland, mucilaginous taste. The leaves contain mucilage of unknown composition and tannins, the flowers the anthocyanin pigment malvin. Like other mucilaginous drugs these have a soothing, anti-inflammatory and softening action.

They are used internally in macerated form or as a component of herbal teas for the relief of cough and in inflammation of the upper respiratory passages. Externally, it is used as an emollient, and in baths and gargles, in the same way as Marsh Mallow.

Today the only sources of the drug are plants grown in Belgium, France, Germany and the countries of south-eastern and eastern Europe.

1. *Part of the stem with flowers and leaves*
2. *Fruit*

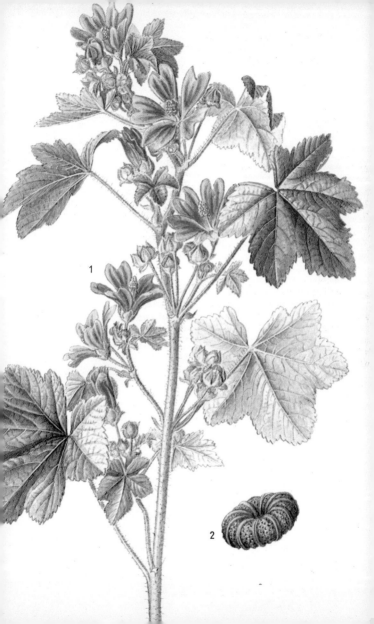

1

2

Marrubium vulgare L.

Labiatae

White Horehound

This is a perennial herb which flowers from June to September and has a local, sometimes quite abundant, distribution on dry pasture land, in waste places and by roadsides from lowland to foothill elevations in warmer climates. It is most probably indigenous to the area extending from the Mediterranean to central Asia, and is established in central and northern Europe, and North and South America.

The top parts *(Herba marrubii albi)* are collected for medicinal use. These are cut during the flowering stage and dried in thin layers in the shade. When dried by artificial heat the temperature must not exceed 40° C. The drug is faintly aromatic and has a bitter flavour. It contains a bitter principle (marrubin), tannins, an undetermined essential oil and mucilage. Marrubin stimulates the appetite and has an expectorant action in bronchitis. It is also believed to correct irregular and rapid heart action.

It is used in the form of an infusion in diseases of the respiratory passages and digestive organs, chiefly the stomach, intestines and gall bladder. The effects, however, are often slight and non-specific. Today it is used mainly as a home remedy.

Formerly the drug was only gathered wild but now it is also cultivated to a limited extent. This medicinal plant has been in use for centuries, even perhaps in ancient Egypt.

Flowering plant

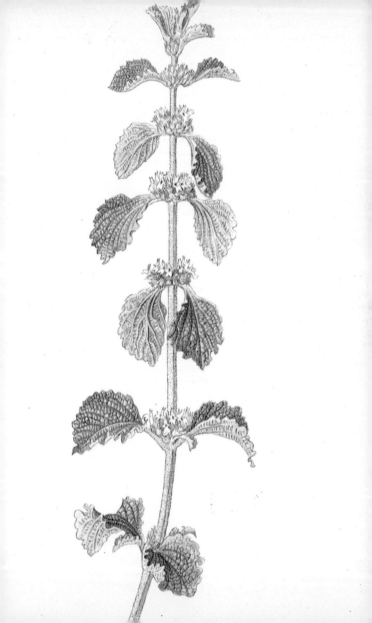

Matricaria chamomilla L. *(M. recutita* L.)

Chamomile

This annual herb, flowering from May to September, often has a second flowering period. It is locally abundant in fields, waste places and at roadsides from lowland to foothill elevations, chiefly in warmer climates. It is most probably a native of the region extending from south-eastern Europe to south-western Asia. It has been cultivated since ancient times, often escaping and becoming established in the wild. The range of distribution covers almost the whole of Europe and large parts of Asia. It was introduced with shipments of seed grain to the Atlantic states of North America and to Australia.

The flower heads *(Flos chamomillae vulgaris)* are collected for the drug market. The quality of the drug depends on when it is gathered. This should be done in dry, sunny weather when about half the flowers are wide open but have not yet begun to droop. Flower heads past their prime easily disintegrate and do not produce a good quality crude drug. The flowers are collected by hand or with a special comb and the stalks should not exceed 2 centimetres in length. They are dried in thin layers in the shade or in drying rooms with artificial heat at temperatures not exceeding 40° C. The drug is highly aromatic and has a bitter spicy taste. It contains sometimes even more than 1 per cent of an essential oil of which blue chamazulene and probably bisabolol, also, are the most medicinally effective constituents. They reduce temperature, and are disinfectant and antispasmodic in action. Subsidiary substances also stimulate the secretion of the sweat glands. The drug is generally used in the form of an infusion both internally and externally. Internally, it is chiefly used in digestive disorders, even in infants, as a component of herbal teas promoting the flow of gastric secretions and bile and in the treatment of colds. Externally, use is made of the anti-inflammatory action of the essential oil on skin and mucous membranes in douches, compresses and baths. Chamomile is also of importance in medicinal cosmetic preparations which make use both of the drug and the essential oil. Because collection in the wild is not sufficient to fulfill the demand, Chamomile is cultivated as a field crop and bred selectively not only for better quality but also larger plant growth to permit gathering by mechanical means.

1. *Flowering plant*
2. *Vertical section through the flower head*
   (the hollow base of the receptacle is characteristic)

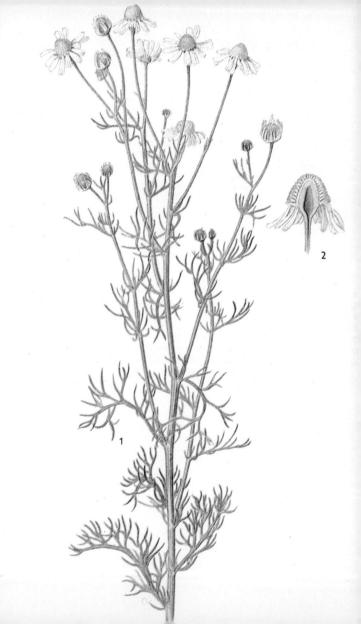

Melissa officinalis L.

Common Balm

This is a perennial herb which flowers from June to August, and is indigenous to the area extending from the Mediterranean through the Caucasus to Iran and south-west Siberia. It has become established in the wild in countries bordering the Mediterranean and southern alpine valleys where it grows in hedgerows, alongside walls, in vineyards and waste places from lowland to hilly country. It is cultivated in the temperate regions of the Northern Hemisphere, both in gardens and as a field crop, for medicinal use, and as a kitchen herb and bee plant; sometimes it escapes and grows wild for a time. *Melissa officinalis* is the species grown most frequently. In the Mediterranean region it has been known since ancient times. It was introduced north of the Alps during the Middle Ages when it was cultivated in monastery gardens.

The parts collected for the drug market are the leaves *(Folium melissae)* and aerial parts *(Herba melissae)*, gathered before the flowering period, usually in June and July, in dry weather. The top parts are cut off above the ground and the leaves stripped. They are dried in thin layers in the shade as rapidly as possible, or in drying rooms by artificial heat at temperatures not exceeding 40° C. Because the crude drug easily turns brown it must not be crushed or turned unnecessarily. It has a lemon odour and pleasant spicy taste. It is stored in closed tins and should not be kept for more than a year. The fresh plant contains about 0.1 per cent of an essential oil, but because of its volatile and unstable nature the amount in the drug rapidly decreases. In addition the drug contains about 5 per cent of tannins and a bitter principle. Its effects are systemically soothing. It relaxes spasms accompanying neurogenic agitation and disorders of the digestive system of similar aetiology.

Internally, it is used in combination with other drugs as an infusion or tincture to treat agitation, insomnia, irritability, digestive disorders and increased heart rate. Externally, it is used as a bath preparation and in anti-rheumatic ointments. The fresh shoots and drug are used to flavour fish and meat dishes and in salads. It is also an essential ingredient in certain liqueurs such as chartreuse.

1. *Flowering plant*
2. *Detail of flower*

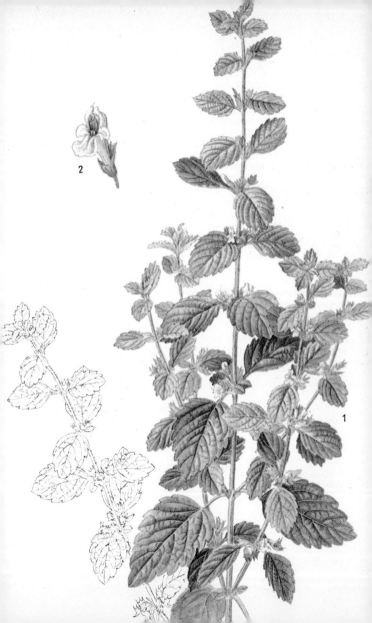

Mentha × *piperita* L.

Labiatae

(= *M. aquatica* L. × *M. spicata* (L.) HUDS.)

Peppermint

This is a perennial herb which flowers from June to August. It is a hybrid of unknown geographical origin described in the late seventeenth century by the British botanist J. Ray. This hybrid is supposed to be the origin of all Peppermint varieties cultivated at the present time. It is widely cultivated in Europe, southern and eastern Asia, North and South America and Australia, chiefly in the varieties *piperita* and *citrata* (EHRH.) BRIQ. It is often found wild but does not become permanently established.

The parts collected for medicinal use are the leaves *(Folium menthae piperitae)* or non-flowering shoots *(Herba menthae piperitae)*, free of peppermint rust *(Puccinia menthae* PERS.*)* and damage by insect pests. These are gathered before the flowering period and quickly dried in the shade or by artificial heat at temperatures not exceeding 40° C. The best method of storage is in cartons or sacks; plastic containers are not suitable because they absorb the essential oil. The drug has an agreeable menthol odour and a cooling, pungent taste. It contains up to 2 per cent of an essential oil which has more than 50 per cent menthol. The drug also contains tannins and bitter principles. It promotes digestion and the secretion of bile, and relieves flatulence and cramps.

The drug is used internally in the form of an infusion or as a component of herbal teas in intestinal and gastric diseases, flatulence, gall bladder disorders and spasms, and externally as a bath preparation in skin rashes of nervous aetiology. The essential oil isolated from it is a component of many medicinal preparations, and has a strong stimulating action on bile secretion as well as an antispasmodic and anti-inflammatory effect. It is also used as a flavouring and aromatic agent in toothpastes and mouthwashes, as well as in liqueurs and in confectionery. Both the drug and essential oil are obtained from cultivated plants — mainly the British cultivar Mitcham or the German cultivar Multimentha. However, other peppermint species, which are named after their geographical source, are also grown.

Flowering plant

158

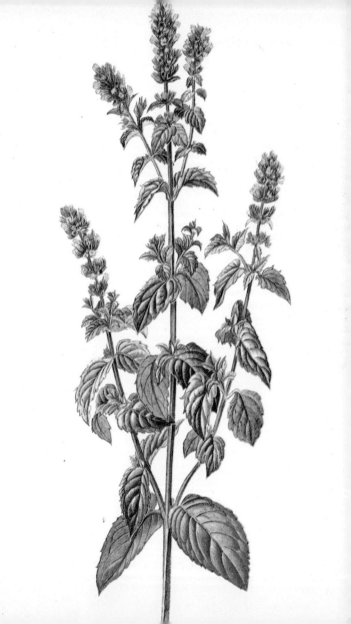

Menyanthes trifoliata L.

Menyanthaceae

Buckbean, Bogbean

This perennial herb flowers from May to June — in mountain areas in August — and is fairly common in swampy meadows, marshes and peat bogs, in ditches and ponds and at the edge of lakes from lowland to mountain elevations. In some places it is the dominant plant in shallow water. It is distributed in the temperate regions of the Northern Hemisphere (as far north as Iceland, and in northern Siberia on the Anadyr River at about latitude 70° N), eastward to Japan, south to the Himalayas and in North America along the Rocky Mountains south to California.

The leaves *(Folium trifolii fibrini)* with short petioles are collected for medicinal use during the flowering stage from May to June. These are laid out to dry in thin layers in a well-ventilated place, after which any leaves that have turned brown must be removed. Artificial heat must not exceed a temperature of 50° C. The drug is odourless and has a strong bitter taste. It contains a glycoside, tannins and flavone compounds. It increases the flow of gastric secretions and has a generally tonic effect.

The drug is used internally either as a powder, or as an infusion or extract, and in herbal tea mixtures to regulate liver and gall bladder function and to stimulate the appetite. It has the same uses as Gentian root and the flowering shoots of Centaury. It is collected only in the wild. Partial cultivation in natural sites seems to be promising.

Flowering plant

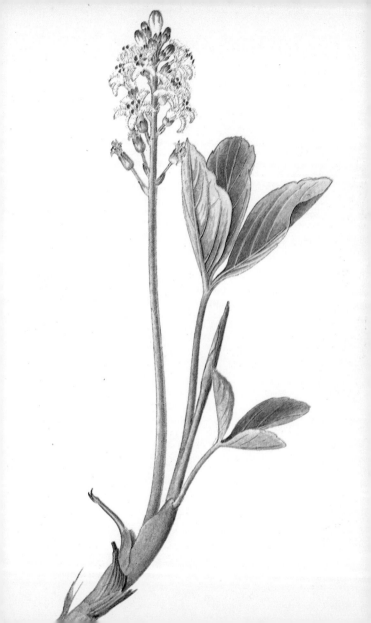

Ocimum basilicum L.

Labiatae

Basil

This is an annual herb, flowering from June to September, and believed by some to be indigenous only to the area from the Middle East to Iran, while others think it to be native to southern Asia or Africa. It has been grown as a medicinal plant or flavouring agent in warmer climates throughout the world for centuries. Sometimes it temporarily grows wild.

The parts collected for the drug market are the flowering shoots *(Herba basilici)* which are cut off several centimetres above the ground and dried either in the shade in a well-ventilated place or by artificial heat at a temperature not exceeding 45° C. The drug has an agreeable spicy odour. It should be stored in tightly closed containers. The active principle is an essential oil which is distilled from the fresh shoots. The yields are about 0.1 per cent.

The drug is used internally as an infusion in digestive disorders and diseases caused by chilling. It promotes gastric function, stimulates the appetite, relieves flatulence and also has an expectorant action. Externally it has a healing effect and is used in compresses and in baths. Besides pharmacy it is used in the food industry to flavour vinegar, mustard and pickled vegetables. Basil oil is also used in perfumery as are the oils of other species of Basil such as *O. gratissimum* L.

The plant is cultivated in North Africa, southern, central and eastern Asia, in the subtropical and tropical regions of America, and in parts of Europe, chiefly in Spain, France and Germany, where it has been grown since the twelfth century.

Flowering plant

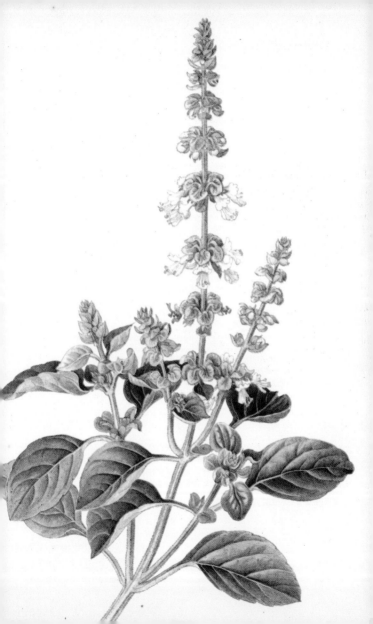

Ononis spinosa L.

Papilionaceae

Restharrow

This is a perennial herb, which flowers from June to September and has a scattered distribution on rough grassland, dry sunny slopes, at the edges of fields and at roadsides from lowland to foothill elevations in warmer climates, chiefly on limestone substrates. It is distributed over practically the whole of Europe, with the exception of the southern, northern and north-eastern areas and alpine regions, and in western Asia (except Arabia) and North Africa.

The active principles are extracted from the root *(Radix ononidis)* which is gathered mainly in the autumn. After cleaning it is dried rapidly at temperatures not exceeding 45° C. The smell of the crude drug is reminiscent of sweet wood and it is biting and sweetish to the tongue. It contains a small amount of an essential oil of unknown composition, glycosides, and other little investigated substances. It has a diuretic action as well as acting as an expectorant in catarrh of the upper respiratory passages.

It is used internally as an infusion and as a component of herbal tea mixtures in the treatment of metabolic disorders, cystitis and rheumatic diseases; externally, it is used in baths for the treatment of chronic skin diseases.

The collection of roots of wild plants is difficult and for that reason Restharrow is now cultivated as a field crop, the roots of two- to three-year growths being harvested by ploughing. It is grown and bred principally in the USSR. Other species besides *Ononis spinosa* L., chiefly those without spines, are also used medicinally.

1. *Root*
2. *Flowering branch*

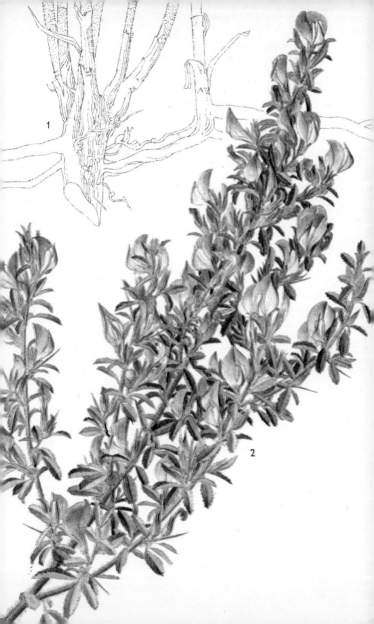

Origanum vulgare L.

Wild Marjoram, Oregano

This is a perennial herb, which flowers from July to September and grows fairly freely on sunny slopes, in dry meadows and clearings, in thickets and copses from lowland to mountain elevations, chiefly in warmer climates. It is distributed throughout the greater part of Europe and the Middle East, in Iran and the area extending to the Himalayas, but is absent from most of the islands in the Mediterranean. It was introduced into the Far East and is also found as a cultivated plant in North America.

The parts collected for the drug market are the flowering shoots (*Herba origani vulgaris*), which are cut and dried in thin layers in the shade or at temperatures not exceeding 45° C. The drug has an agreeable aromatic odour and spicy, somewhat astringent taste. It contains about 0.5 per cent of an essential oil, specially bred cultivars even more. The composition of the oil depends on such factors as the species, the plant's geographical source, and the time when it was collected. The drug also contains bitter principles and tannins. The various constituents aid digestion, relax spasms and have a disinfectant effect in intestinal disorders, besides which they also exert an expectorant action and reduce inflammation.

The drug is used internally as an infusion in digestive disorders. Its disinfectant and germicidal effects are used in heavy coughs and diseases of the repiratory passages. External application — in the form of gargles, inhalants and baths — is also recommended. Marjoram is a common kitchen herb and is used by the food industry to flavour salamis, sausages and salads; it is also used in cosmetics, especially in soap. A volatile oil distilled from the herb on a commercial scale has similar uses.

Today cultivation of the type plant, as well as other species important for the composition of their essential oil, is becoming widespread. In Mediterranean countries, however, it is still collected wild.

1. *Flowering plant*
2. *Detail of flower*

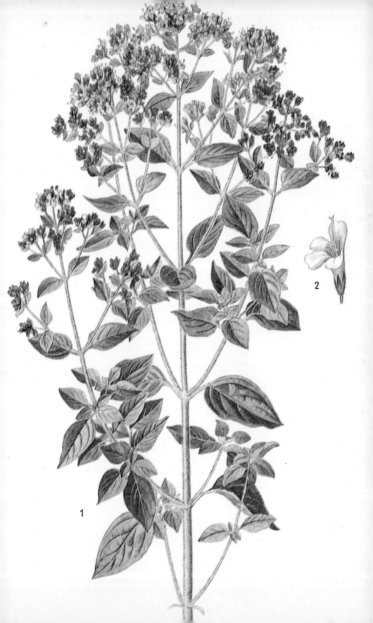

1
2

Papaver somniferum L.

Papaveraceae

Opium Poppy

This annual herb, which flowers from July to August, has been cultivated for centuries. The type plant is considered to be the Mediterranean poppy *P. setigerum*. The Opium Poppy is most probably a native of the Middle East but it is now cultivated in the temperate regions of the Northern Hemisphere for its oily seeds, as a medicinal plant and for the production of opium from the Mediterranean countries to subtropical Asia, as far as China and Japan. Its cultivation in Eurasia is believed to have spread from east to west, not vice versa.

The raw material for pharmaceutic purposes is the milky exudation obtained by making incisions into unripe capsules (opium) and the empty, dry capsules *(Fructus papaveris maturus)*. The principal sources of opium are Turkey (Asia Minor), India, the USSR and China. The dried capsules are a pharmaceutical raw material in many European countries. Both the crude opium and dry capsules contain extremely toxic alkaloids, more than twenty of which have been isolated to date. Opium contains about 12 per cent of morphine, the dry capsules far less (0.3—1.2 per cent). The most important opium alkaloids are morphine, narcotine, papaverine, codeine, thebaine and narceine. Morphine reduces sensitivity to pain even in those cases where standard medicines are ineffective and has a general depressant action on the nerve centres. Codeine increases the pain-killing effects of numerous medicines and suppresses the desire to cough. Papaverine relaxes even marked contractions of smooth muscle. In pharmacy the opium alkaloids are a component part of numerous commercial preparations. Morphine and crude opium are subject to international narcotic laws and therefore their production and the medicines made from them are under strict medical and official supervision.

1. *Top of a flowering plant with a bud*
2. *Unripe capsules, one of them with drops of milky latex exuding from the incision made in its wall*

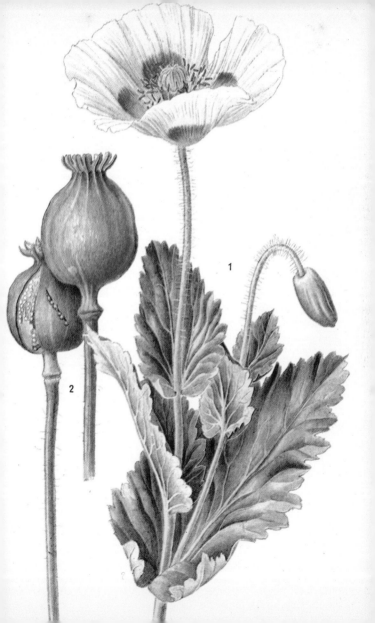

Pastinaca sativa L.

Wild Parsnip

A biennial herb flowering from July to August, Wild Parsnip grows fairly freely, and is sometimes locally abundant, on grassy waste land, at the roadside and in hedgerows from lowland to foothill elevations. It is distributed throughout most of Europe and western Asia. However, it is completely absent from some areas. The wild plant is abundant in central Europe, introduced and established in North America, Uruguay, Australia and New Zealand. Cultivars which differ in the shape of the thick fleshy root belong to the variety *sativa hortensis* EHRH.

The active principles are extracted from the root *(Radix pastinaceae)*, gathered in July and August, and sometimes also from the fruit *(Fructus pastinaceae)*, collected in September. The temperature when drying must not exceed 40° C. The drug has an aromatic odour and sharp taste. Because this is a plant which in damp or sunny weather may cause an allergic skin reaction it should not be collected by those who are susceptible. All collectors should protect their skin when gathering this herb. The active principles of the drug are furocoumarins, which when exposed to light cause photodermatoses. The fruits contain more than 1 per cent, the roots about 0.2 per cent of these active principles. Besides furocoumarins, they also include an essential oil which has not been thoroughly investigated as yet.

The drugs have a diuretic as well as soothing effect and also stimulate the appetite. They are used internally in the form of an infusion in loss of appetite and in urinary disorders. Today Parsnip is used primarily as a vegetable which tastes a little like a cross between Carrot and Parsley. The drug can be obtained from vegetable crops when needed.

1. *Root*
2. *Part of a flowering plant*
3. *Detail of flower*
4. *Detail of fruit*

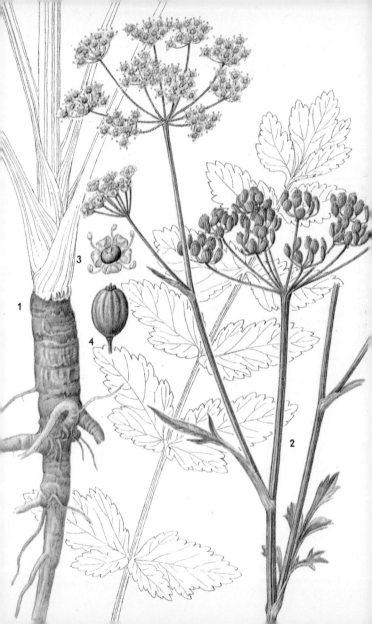

Petroselinum crispum (P. MILL.) NYM.
(P. hortense HOFFM.*)*

Umbelliferae

Parsley

Parsley is a biennial herb which flowers from June to July, and is probably indigenous to the Mediterranean region; it is cultivated throughout the world as a culinary herb (var. *vulgare* NOIS. DANERT — with smooth leaf margins and var. *crispum* — with crinkled leaf margins) or sometimes as a root vegetable (var. *radicosum* BAILEY). It often grows wild by roadsides and on waste land.

The parts of the plant used for medicinal purposes are the roots *(Radix petroselini)* and fruits *(Fructus petroselini)*, and occasionally the aerial parts *(Herba petroselini)* also. The roots are gathered as late as possible in the autumn or in the spring of the second year's growth, cut in pieces and dried at a temperature not exceeding 40° C. The fruits are cut off and left to ripen on large sheets of canvas, after which the seeds are separated by threshing and then cleaned. The drug has a characteristic spicy odour and sweetish taste, due to its content of an essential oil. The seeds contain up to 7 per cent of the essential oil, the roots about 0.1 per cent and the leaves up to 0.3 per cent. Small medicinal doses of the drug aid digestion, have a strong diuretic action and relieve flatulence. Larger doses, however, cause congestion of the membrane lining the uterus and therefore must not be used during pregnancy. Large doses of the oil have stupefying effects.

The drugs are used internally as an infusion, as a component of herbal tea mixtures or specifics in urinary diseases and inflammation of the prostate gland. A volatile oil can be distilled from the seeds, roots and green parts which, in addition to its use in medicine, is also used as a flavouring in the food industry. Fresh parsley is a popular garnish and flavouring in soups, salads and all kinds of other dishes. It has been grown for centuries.

The only source of the drug is the cultivated plant.

1. *Root*
2. *Part of a flowering plant*
3. *Detail of flower*
4. *Detail of leaf*
5. *Detail of fruit*

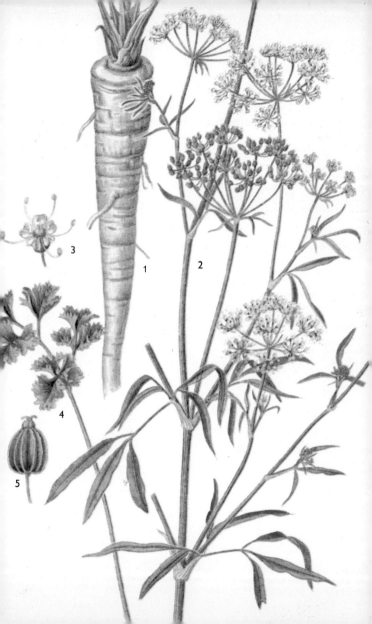

1
2
3
4
5

Pimpinella saxifraga L.

Umbelliferae

Burnet Saxifrage

This is a perennial herb flowering from June to October. It grows abundantly in dry meadows and pastures, at the edges of fields and on railway banks, at the roadside and in waste places from lowland to subalpine elevations, occasionally also at alpine altitudes. It is distributed throughout most of Europe, excepting the southernmost regions, and in the Middle East and western Siberia. It has been introduced and become established in North America, and temporarily in New Zealand also.

It is the roots *(Radix pimpinellae)* which are collected for medicinal purposes, generally in September and October. After cleaning they are dried naturally, if possible; if artificial heat has to be used, then the temperature should not exceed 45° C. The drug has a distinct odour and a sweetish, pungent flavour and should be stored in tightly closed containers to protect it from damp. It contains about 0.4 per cent of an essential oil and tannins. Its action is diuretic; it also increases the flow of digestive secretions and alleviates respiratory diseases.

It is used internally as an infusion in catarrh of the respiratory passages, flatulence and disorders of gastric secretion, and in kidney and urinary diseases. Externally, it is used as a gargle and as a bath preparation. In mediaeval times Burnet Saxifrage was believed to ward off the plague. Young leaves are used in salads and to flavour sauces. The essential oil is used in liqueurs.

Pimpinella nigra (P. MILL.) GAUD., which is sometimes used instead of *Pimpinella saxifraga* L., contains a blue essential oil supposedly rich in chamazulene, which is mostly obtained from the root. The drug has similar applications.

The drug is collected only in the wild, although it was cultivated in Germany as a medicinal plant as early as the beginning of the second half of the sixteenth century.

1. *Flowering plant*
2. *Detail of flower*
3. *Leaf*
4. *Root*

174

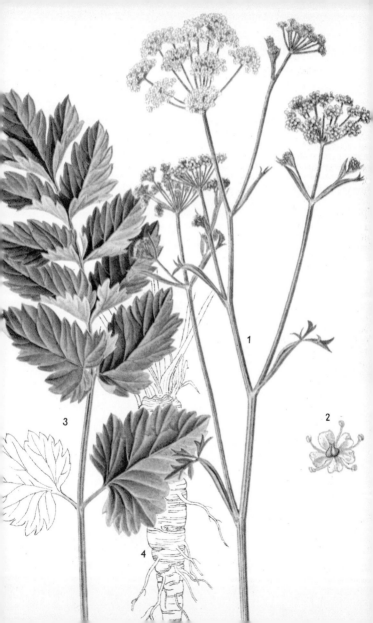

Plantago lanceolata L.

Ribwort

This is a perennial herb which flowers from May to September and grows freely in grassy places on basic neutral soils from lowland to mountain elevations. It is distributed throughout most of Europe (including Iceland) and in western Asia as far east as the western Himalayas. It has been introduced into eastern Siberia and the Far East, North Africa, Ethiopia, Ceylon, Norway and South America, Australia and New Zealand.

The leaves *(Folium plantaginis lanceolatae)* are used for extraction of the active principles; they are collected from June to August and dried rapidly in thin layers by artificial heat at temperatures not exceeding 50° C. They must be gathered and dried with care because if crushed they turn brown or even black. The drug is odourless and has a faintly bitter, astringent taste. It contains mucilage, tannins, a glycoside and other substances of which there is at present little chemical knowledge. It exerts a beneficial effect in diseases of the upper respiratory passages caused by chilling. It is a popular home remedy for healing wounds, especially those which have become infected.

It is used internally in the form of an infusion, as a component of herbal teas for chest colds, and in syrups and lozenges in disorders associated with chilling. Externally the juice of the fresh leaves is applied to wounds for its anti-inflammatory and healing properties.

Plantain is beginning to be cultivated for medicinal purposes because the collection of wild plants is unable to meet the demand. Also cultivated in the Mediterranean region are the species *Plantago psyllium* L. and *P. indica* L.; with these herbs it is the seeds which are collected for the drug, which contains as much as 10 per cent of mucilage.

Flowering plant

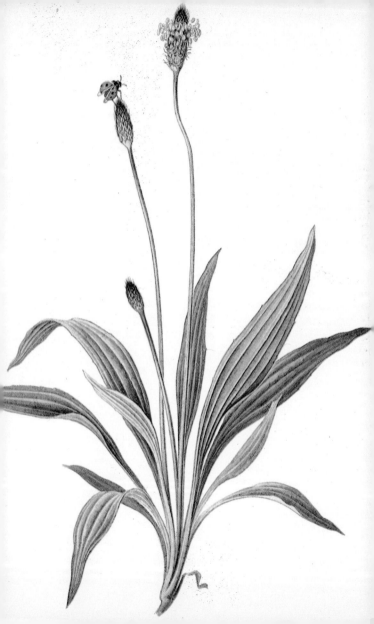

Polygonum hydropiper L.

Polygonaceae

Water Pepper

This is an annual herb which flowers from June to October and is generally distributed in damp and wet places and in shallow water in ponds and ditches. It acts as an indicator of the increasing dampness of the substrate, and is found from lowland to foothill, and occasionally at mountain elevations. It is distributed in the temperate and southern regions of Eurasia (in Asia as far south as Ceylon and Indonesia) and in North Africa.

The aerial parts *(Herba polygoni hydropiperis)*, are collected for medicinal purposes, cut during the flowering stage from June to September and dried naturally in a well-ventilated place or in drying rooms at temperatures not exceeding 40° C. The drug is odourless and has a peppery taste. Sometimes fresh shoots are used. It contains an essential oil with volatile fatty acids and camphor-like substances, anthraquinones, tannins and flavones. It checks bleeding and relieves menstrual pains. The astringent effect is produced by the tannins.

The drug is used internally as an infusion or in herbal teas to check strong menstrual discharge and hemorrhoidal bleeding. Externally, it is sometimes used in the treatment of suppurating arthritis.

The drug is collected only in the wild. In ancient times the ripe seed vessels were used as a substitute for black pepper.

1. *Flowering top*
2. *Fruit*

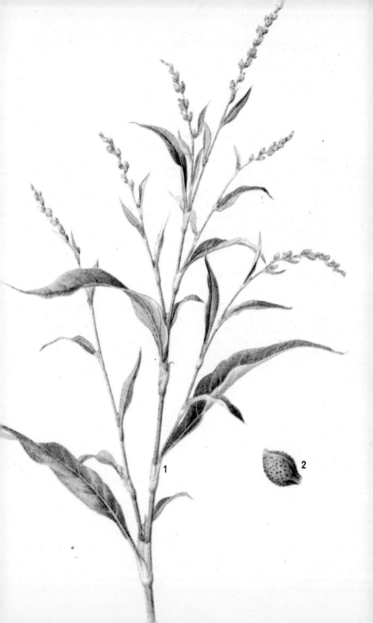

1

2

Potentilla erecta (L.) HAMPE
(P. tormentilla NECK.*)*

Rosaceae

Common Tormentil

This is a perennial herb, flowering from June to October, which grows freely in meadows, woods and heaths from lowland to alpine elevations. It is distributed in Europe with the exceptions of Sicily, Albania and Greece, all the way to western Siberia, which marks the boundary of its continuous range.

The rhizomes *(Radix tormentillae)* are collected for medicinal purposes either in spring (March-April) or autumn (September-October). They are thoroughly cleaned and laid out to dry naturally in thin layers in a well-ventilated spot, the drying process being completed by artificial heat at temperatures not exceeding 70° C. The drug's chief constituents are catechol tannins (17—22 per cent) which are gradually converted into the dark-red tannins called phlobaphenes. Besides tannins, glycosides and organic acids are also believed to be present. The drug exerts an astringent and anti-inflammatory effect.

It is used internally, generally as a decoction or as a component of herbal tea mixtures in the treatment of diarrhoea, and chronic and acute gastric and intestinal catarrh. Externally, it is used as a decoction and tincture applied to inflamed gums, and as a mouthwash in stomatitis. It is a component of certain pharmaceutical preparations used in the external treatment of hemorrhoids and frostbite.

The drug is collected only in the wild.

Flowering plant

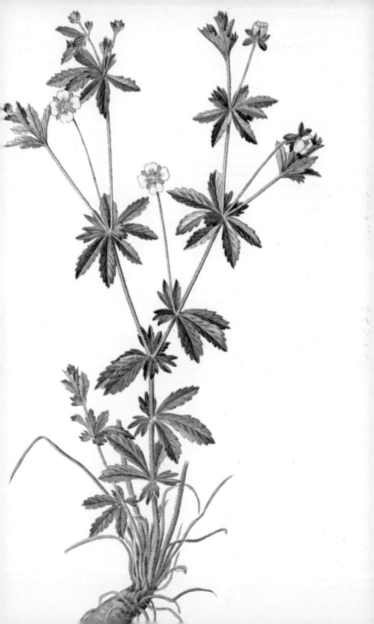

Primula veris L.

Cowslip

This is a perennial herb flowering from April to May and growing in meadows and pastures on basic and especially calcareous soils, from lowland to foothill elevations; it is locally abundant. The range of distribution embraces the temperate regions of Eurasia. In eastern Siberia it is believed to occur only as an introduced plant.

The parts serving for extraction of the active principles are the roots *(Radix primulae)* or flowers *(Flos primulae)*. The former are gathered from March to May, thoroughly washed and dried at a temperature not exceeding 45° C. The flowers (including the calyx) are collected from April to May and are dried naturally. The drug smells like Anise and has a very pungent taste. It contains up to 10 per cent of saponins and glycosides which yield an essential oil known as primula camphor. The roots yield an average of 0.085 per cent and the flowers 0.01 per cent of the oil. The active principles have an expectorant effect in inflammation of the upper respiratory passages.

They are used internally as a decoction, as a tea or in commercial pharmaceutical preparations for the treatment of respiratory diseases, primarily as an expectorant.

The drug is collected only in the wild, attempts at cultivation having been unprofitable to date. The active principles may also be obtained from Oxlip *(Primula elatior* [L.] HILL*)*, which grows in the same type of localities as Cowslip but often at higher altitudes. It does not occur in warmer climates. The range of distribution includes Europe, although it is not found south of the Alps, and the area extending from the Caucasus through northern Iran to the Altai.

Flowering plant

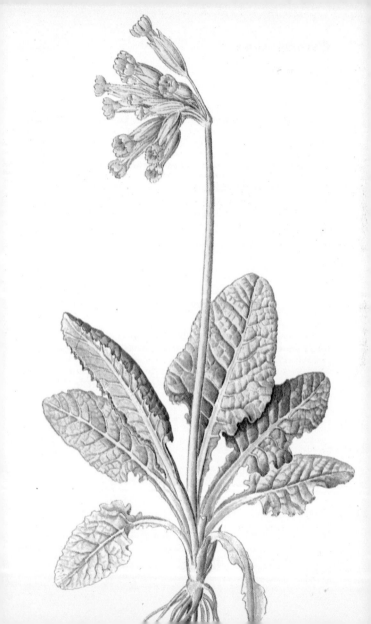

Quercus robur L.

Fagaceae

Common Oak

This is a deciduous tree, flowering from May to June, which is characteristic of heavy and basic soils (clays and loams). It grows fairly abundantly to abundantly in pure stands or mixed with other deciduous and coniferous trees, in meadowland and hedgerows from lowland to foothill, occasionally even at mountain elevations. It is found in all but the extreme north and south of Europe to the Urals and Caucasus.

The young bark without the outer corky layer *(Cortex quercus)* is collected for medicinal purposes. It is peeled from branches cut from the tree, best of all in spring. The smooth, grey-brown 'mirror bark', which still has a silvery sheen, is of great value. Older, cracked bark is not collected at all. It is generally dried in the sun or by artificial heat at a temperature not exceeding 50° C. The crude drug is up to 2 millimetres thick, curled inward like a split tube. It has a characteristic tannic odour and bitter, astringent taste. When stored for a long time the quantity of water soluble tannins is reduced and the efficacy of the drug is decreased. The bark contains 10—20 per cent of tannins and other subsidiary substances. It has a strong astringent, anti-inflammatory and costive action. Large doses, however, cause retching.

It is used internally only to a limited extent as a decoction in the treatment of gastro-intestinal catarrh and diarrhoea, externally as an extract and as a decoction in compresses and baths for the treatment of frostbite and rashes, to inhibit excessive sweating, and in combination with Chamomile in the treatment of hemorrhoids. The acorns were formerly used as an antidote to poisoning and diarrhoea. The drug is little used medicinally, however, its chief importance today being in the tanning industry for the processing of leather.

Cortex quercus is also obtained from the Durmast Oak *(Q. petraea* [MATTUSCHKA] LIEBL. [*Q. sessilis* EHRH.]*)*, which grows fairly commonly on rocky soils with the Common Oak in mixed woods from lowland to foothill elevations. It is widespread in Europe from the Iberian Peninsula to the Vologda-Podolsk region in the USSR, south to Albania and north to western Norway.

1. *Flowering branch*   3. *Male flowers*
2. *Female flowers*   4. *Branch with acorns*

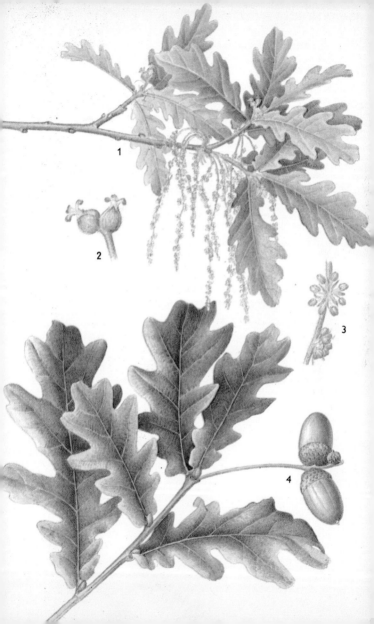

Rheum palmatum L.   Polygonaceae

Rhubarb

This is a perennial herbaceous plant, flowering from June to July, which is indigenous to north-west China and north-east Tibet. It is grown chiefly in the USSR and in Germany. It has been cultivated in European gardens as an ornamental plant since 1763.

The parts collected for the drug market are the rhizomes (*Rhizoma rhei*) of second- and third-year growths gathered in the autumn. After being cleaned, peeled and cut into smaller pieces they are threaded on strings and hung up to dry either naturally or by artificial heat in drying rooms at temperatures not exceeding 50° C. The drug has a characteristic odour and bitter flavour. Besides tannins it contains about 10 per cent of free as well as bound anthraquinones, which are the chief active principles. However, it must not contain the glycoside rhaponticin, which has hormonal effects and is present in the rhizomes of the species *R. rhabarbarum* L. and *R. rhaponticum* L. In small doses of up to 0.5 grams the chief action is exerted by the tannins and is costive, whereas in doses of 1—3 grams the chief action is exerted by the anthraquinones which have a cathartic effect.

The drug is used internally as a powder or as a specific in chronic constipation, gastric and intestinal catarrh and as an agent stimulating the appetite. It must not be used by persons suffering from kidney stones or urinary gravel.

The drug is collected only in the wild, the chief source of European supply being China. Attempts are being made to cultivate it in Europe. The related species *R. rhabarbarum* L. has long been grown in gardens as a food plant.

1. *Rhizome*
2. *Part of the stem with flowers and fruits*
3. *Detail of fruit*

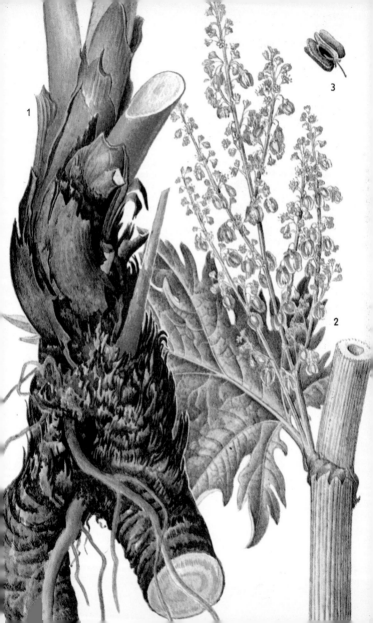

Rosmarinus officinalis L.

Labiatae

Rosemary

This evergreen shrub flowers from April to May and grows abundantly in the maquis of the Mediterranean coast, where it has been widely cultivated since ancient times. It has become fully established in some parts of this area. North of the Alps it is grown chiefly as a potted garden plant, although in certain parts with mild winters it is possible to grow it in the ground. The species comprises several varieties, those found in Algeria being sometimes described as independent species.

The parts collected for the drug market are the leaves *(Folium rosmarini)* stripped from plants in summer. These are then dried either in thin layers in a shaded, well-ventilated spot or else by artificial heat at a temperature not exceeding 40° C. The drug smells somewhat like camphor and has an aromatic flavour. It contains 1—2 per cent of an essential oil and tannins. It increases the flow of gastric secretions, bile and urine; it has disinfectant properties and irritant effects; in larger doses it is toxic and causes convulsions and delusions.

The drug is now generally used only in popular home remedies. It is administered internally in the form of an infusion both as a tonic and to increase the flow of bile and urine. Use is made of Rosemary oil in ointments and liniments to alleviate pain in rheumatism of the muscles or joints and in neuritis. The drug is important as a source of the essential oil used chiefly in perfumes and insect repellents.

The drug is collected only in the wild, the chief sources of supply being Spain, Yugoslavia, Italy, France and countries on the coast of North Africa.

1. *Flowering branches*
2. *Detail of flower*

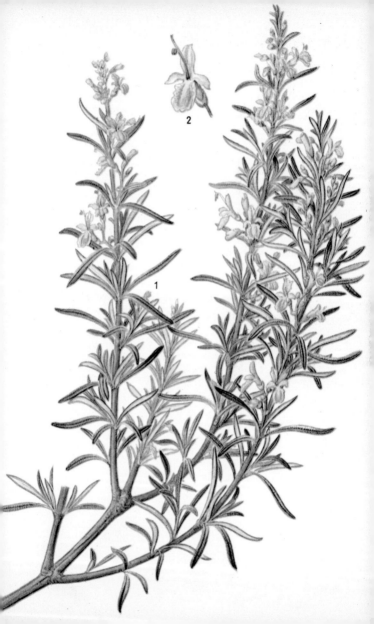

1

2

Rubia tinctorum L.

Madder Root

Madder Root is a perennial herb flowering from June to August. It is indigenous to the Mediterranean countries of Europe and Turkey, and was formerly widely cultivated in France, the Netherlands and central Europe where it often became wild. Remnants of its cultivation are found only in Alsace, where the growing of Madder Root was introduced from other parts of France — the natural colouring matter alizarin was used to dye the trousers of the French infantry red and for the same purpose in the case of Turkish fezes. Now it is cultivated solely for medicinal purposes in Europe and central Asia. It has been grown in the Mediterranean region since ancient times.

The roots *(Radix rubiae)* of this plant are gathered in spring (March to April) or autumn (September to October) from two-year or, exceptionally, three-year growths. They are first cleaned and then dried, generally by artificial heat at temperatures not exceeding 50° C. The drug has a marked odour and a slightly bitter, astringent taste. It contains anthraquinone derivatives as water-soluble pigments, of which the one of greatest therapeutic importance is ruberythric acid.

Its properties prevent the formation of stones in the kidneys and urinary bladder, and have a diuretic, disinfectant and soothing effect. The drug is used internally as a powder, as a decoction, in herbal tea mixtures or as a component of specifics in the treatment of kidney and bladder stones. It has been proved that the active principles cause the disintegration of stones and their consequent elimination in the urine. They also relax muscle tension, thereby aiding the process. Externally the drug is occasionally used in the treatment of abscesses and recalcitrant wounds.

1. *Root*
2. *Flowering part of a plant*

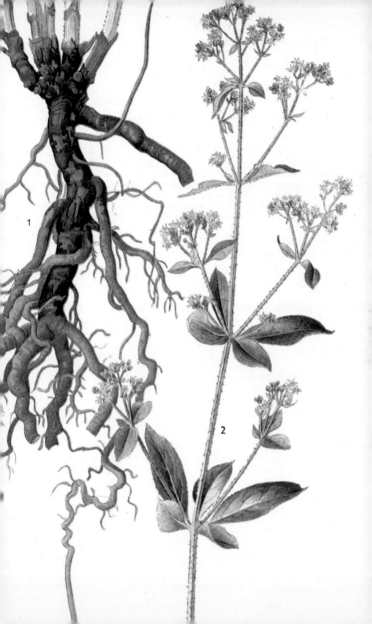

Ruta graveolens L.

Rue

Rue is a perennial herb flowering from June to August. It grows on dry, rocky slopes and limestone screes in Mediterranean Europe. It is an important plant of the Adriatic karst regions and has become fully established in the southern Alps, southern France and Spain.

The tops *(Herba rutae)* are cut during the flowering period and are dried in the shade or by artificial heat at temperatures below 40° C. The drug has a spicy odour and a bitter taste. It should not be gathered by anyone who is liable to allergies. It contains about 0.1 per cent of an essential oil as well as the glycoside rutin, a bitter principle, resin, tannin, furocoumarins and other substances. The drug increases blood flow to the digestive organs and smooth muscle, has abortive and diuretic properties and possesses an anthelmintic effect. Large doses are toxic, causing retching and delusions.

The drug is used as an infusion or in some other form for disorders of the autonomic nervous system. It must only be used under medical supervision and must not be taken during pregnancy. It is used externally in baths in the treatment of skin diseases and suppurating wounds but only in such dosage as will not cause excessive irritation of the skin.

The essential oil recovered from this plant is also used in perfumery. Rue is used in very small amounts as a flavouring agent in meat dishes and sauces, and in combination with Juniper berries, Sage, Thyme and the leaves of the Grape Vine in cooking game.

The drug is collected wild.

Flowering top part

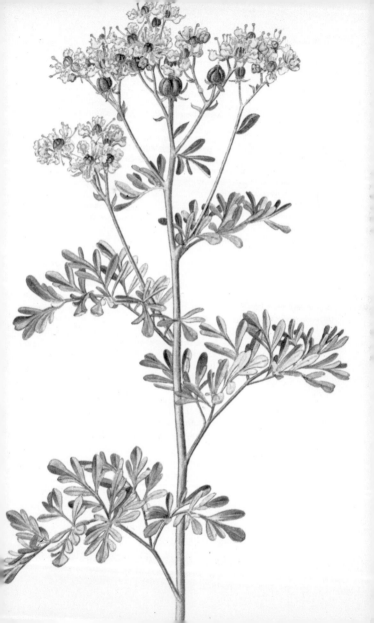

Salvia officinalis L.

Labiatae

Garden Sage

This semi-shrub, flowering from May to July, grows fairly abundantly on dry, sunny slopes and limestone rocks. It is indigenous to the Mediterranean countries of Europe, but it has become established elsewhere in the Mediterranean region and also in southern Germany. It has been commonly cultivated in central Europe as an annual herb since early mediaeval times. It is grown in North America, too.

The active principles are concentrated in the leaves *(Folium salviae)*. The top parts are cut off before the flowering stage in May and June, and the leaves are stripped and dried rapidly at temperatures not exceeding 40° C. The drug is aromatic and may contain more than 2 per cent of an essential oil with over fifty constituents whose proportions vary according to the geographic source and time of collection. In addition it contains tannins, oestrogens and organic acids. It inhibits the growth of bacteria and fungi, lowers the secretion of the sweat glands, exerts a mild diuretic effect, and has anti-inflammatory and astringent properties.

The drug has been used in the form of an infusion or as a component of herbal tea mixtures or specifics to inhibit nocturnal sweating in sufferers from tuberculosis as well as in liver and gall bladder diseases and inflammation of the upper respiratory passages. It can be used as a gargle in stomatitis and in compresses applied to old and recalcitrant wounds. Sage oil, distilled commercially from the drug, is used in pharmacy for the same purposes. The drug and the essential oil are also used to flavour meat dishes, poultry, salads, herb cheeses and vinegar.

The drug is collected chiefly in the wild (Dalmatia, Albania), being cultivated as a field crop only to a limited degree; it is, however, often grown in gardens for culinary use. The eastern Mediterranean region is the home of the closely related *S. tomentosa* P. MILL., but this species is not used as a drug.

Flowering stem

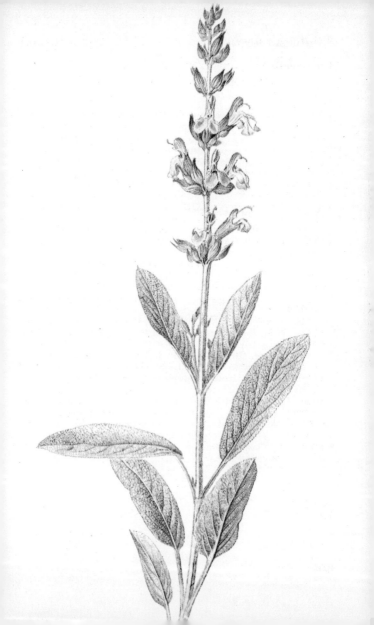

Sambucus nigra L.

Caprifoliaceae

Elderberry

The Elderberry is a tree or shrub flowering from June to July. It grows abundantly at all altitudes in deciduous and riverside woods, in thickets and clearings, also in barren places, alongside walls, fences and buildings. It is distributed throughout most of Europe, Turkey, and perhaps also in western Siberia and North Africa. It is indigenous to the riverside woods of central Europe and is cultivated in some places. It is always found near human habitations.

The parts collected for medicinal use are the flowers *(Flos sambuci)* and fruits *(Fructus sambuci)*. The inflorescences are cut off in dry weather, spread out on nets to wilt, after which the blooms are divested of the stalks and left to dry in the shade. The drug has a strong odour and is sweet and scratchy to the tongue. Fruits are gathered when ripe and dried in the same way as the flowers; they are odourless, sour and astringent. The flowers contain the flavonoid glycoside rutin, an essential oil, tannins, other glycosides, mucilages and organic acids. The fruits contain organic acids, tannins, anthocyanide pigments, a small amount of an essential oil and vitamin C. Both drugs reduce fever, stimulate secretion of the sweat glands and have a beneficial effect on chronic catarrh of the respiratory passages. They furthermore exert a diuretic and antispasmodic action.

The flowers are taken internally in the form of an infusion for fevers caused by chilling, catarrh of the respiratory passages and rheumatism. They can be used as a gargle and as a bath preparation. The juice from the fruits is used internally in the treatment of migraine and neuralgias, and to reduce sensitivity to pain. Tea from elderberries has a beneficial effect in chronic inflammation of the upper respiratory passages. In some regions a tasty and refreshing beverage is made by fermenting the fresh flowers with lemon juice and lemon peel. The fruits are sometimes fermented to make wine.

The drug is collected only in the wild.

1. *Flowering branch*
2. *Fruits*

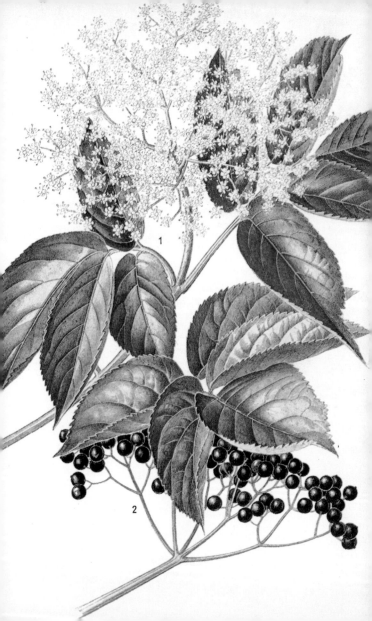

Satureja hortensis L.

Savory

An annual herb flowering from July to September, Savory is indigenous to the eastern Mediterranean and south-west Asia. It grows on rocky slopes, in fields, and alongside highways and railways. It occurs both wild and established elsewhere in the Mediterranean region, in central Europe, India, South Africa and North America. It was probably first cultivated in Italy, and since the ninth century in central Europe also, chiefly in monastery gardens.

The aerial parts *(Herba saturejae)*, including the leaves, or sometimes only the flowering tops are gathered. These are tied in bunches or spread out on wooden frames to dry in the shade or with artificial heat at temperatures below 40° C. The drug is aromatic and pungent, with a taste somewhat reminiscent of pepper, and is stored in tins. It contains 0.8—1.5 per cent of an essential oil, together with tannins, resin, and mucilages. It exerts a carminative action, aids digestion, and has a mild diuretic as well as anthelmintic effect.

It is used internally in the form of an infusion in gastric and intestinal catarrh, and also for its fairly reliable anthelmintic action. The fresh leaves are used chiefly to season beans, salads, cucumbers, fish, meat, salamis and sausages. The drug yields an essential oil used by the food industry.

The drug is collected wild, the chief source of supply being the Mediterranean region, where it is also cultivated to a small extent as in central Europe and other areas. The crude drug from other species such as *S. montana* L. and *S. cuneifolia* TEN. — both from the Mediterranean region — is also used pharmaceutically.

Flowering top part

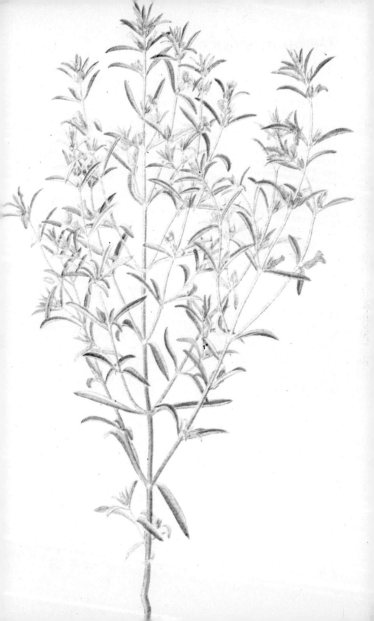

Thymus serpyllum L.

Wild Thyme

This is a semi-shrub or perennial herb, flowering from May to September, with a scattered to abundant distribution on sunny hillsides, pastureland, sandy soil, rocks, in open woods and clearings from lowland to alpine elevations. It is distributed throughout the temperate regions of Eurasia and occurs also in Greenland, Iceland and the Yenisei River region of Siberia. It has become established in North America.

The aerial parts *(Herba serpylli)* are gathered shortly before the flowering stage. The tops with flower buds are cut and dried in the shade or in drying rooms with artificial heat at temperatures up to 40° C. The drug is aromatic and has a slightly bitter, spicy taste. It contains about 0.3 per cent of an essential oil the composition of which depends on the geographic source and other factors. The drug contains flavones, tannins, and bitter principles. It has a beneficial effect in diseases of the upper respiratory tract and in digestive disorders because it relaxes spasms and inhibits flatulence.

It is used internally in the form of an infusion, drops or syrup for irritating coughs and catarrh of the upper respiratory passages as well as for gastro-intestinal disorders. As a bath preparation it is employed in the treatment of suppurating wounds and rheumatism. The drug yields an essential oil that has antiseptic properties — it is used in some gargles, mouthwashes and toothpastes — but is otherwise similar to Thyme oil.

The drug is collected only in the wild and thus generally consists of a combination of several species of *Thymus*.

Flowering plant

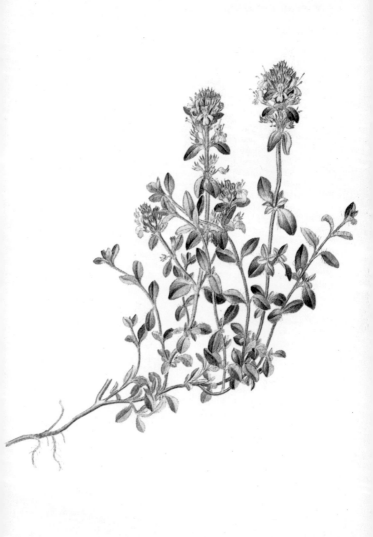

Thymus vulgaris L.   Labiatae

Garden Thyme

Garden Thyme is a semi-shrub, flowering from May to October, growing on rocky ground and in maquis. It is found throughout the European countries bordering the Mediterranean. In the Maritime Alps it occurs at high altitudes. North of the Alps it is cultivated as an annual herb. Thyme has been known as a medicinal plant in the Mediterranean region since ancient times and north of the Alps since the eleventh century.

The aerial parts *(Herba thymi)* are collected for the drug market before the flowering stage and dried in thin layers in a well-ventilated spot. If artifical heat is used then the temperature should not exceed 40° C. After drying, the leaves and flowers are generally stripped from the stems. The drug is pungent and has a pleasantly aromatic flavour. It contains 0.4—0.7 per cent of an essential oil and up to 7 per cent of tannins, bitter principles, flavones and other substances. The composition of the active principles is influenced by the plant's geographic source and, in the case of cultivated growths, the soil nutrients and moisture also. Cultivars have been bred that contain more than 2 per cent of the essential oil. The drug's disinfectant and germicidal effects are most marked in diseases of the upper respiratory passages and of the digestive organs.

It is used internally in the form of an infusion or as a component of herbal tea mixtures, drops and syrups for diseases of the respiratory passages and digestive disorders. It is applied externally in bath preparations, in compresses applied to suppurating wounds, as a gargle and in mouthwashes. Thyme yields an essential oil that is used in pharmacy in the same way as the crude drug. Besides this it is a common kitchen herb of the French cuisine, used in cooking game and certain fish dishes.

The drug is collected wild (the Mediterranean countries, Spain, France) and is also cultivated (Germany, France, Hungary and other countries).

Flowering plant

202

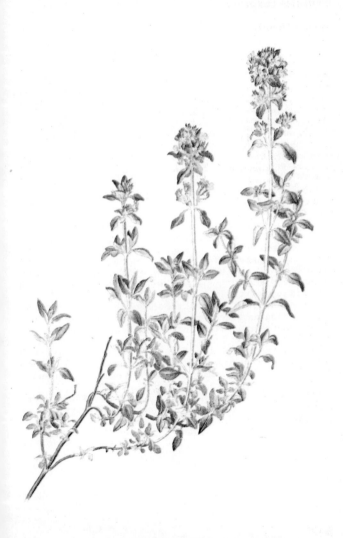

Tilia cordata P. MILL.

Tiliaceae

Small-leaved Lime

A tree — less frequently a shrub — flowering from June to July, the Small-leaved Lime grows fairly abundantly in deciduous or mixed woods, in thickets, on sun-warmed slopes and rocks, and alongside waterways from lowland to foothill elevations. It is a popular species for tree avenues and parks. It is distributed throughout most of Europe, and is cultivated in North America.

The flowers *(Flos tiliae)* — the whole inflorescence including the membranous bract — are collected for medicinal purposes. The blossoms are collected at the beginning of the flowering stage in dry weather and dried in thin layers in the shade in a spot with very good ventilation. If artificial heat is used the temperature should be 40° C. The drug has a faint, honey-like odour and a sweetish taste. It contains about 0.02 per cent of an essential oil from which farnesol has been isolated plus mucilages and flavonoid glycosides; it has been little investigated chemically. The drug exerts a mild diuretic action, stimulates the secretion of the sweat glands, and has an expectorant and antispasmodic effect.

Internally it is used in the form of an infusion or in herbal tea mixtures for treating the effects of chills (mucous congestion of the respiratory passages, cough), as a subsidiary sweat-promoting medicine in influenza, in the treatment of urinary diseases and to stimulate the flow of digestive secretions. Its application is similar to that of Elderberry. Externally it is used as a gargle, in mouthwashes and in baths.

The drug is collected only in the wild. Scarcity of the drug is caused chiefly by the difficulty of collecting and therefore attempts are being made to cultivate limes of shrubby stature, which would be more suitable for this purpose.

Other species of lime, such as the American Lime *(T. americana* L.*)* and Silver Lime *(T. argentea* DESF.*)* are not suited for drug production since they contain substances that cause gastric disorders and nausea. However, the inflorescence of the Large-leaved Lime *(T. platyphyllos* SCOP.*),* growing in similar localities to the Small-leaved Lime and widespread in central and southern Europe, is also used for the drug.

1. *Branch with blossoms*
2. *Fruit with bract*

204

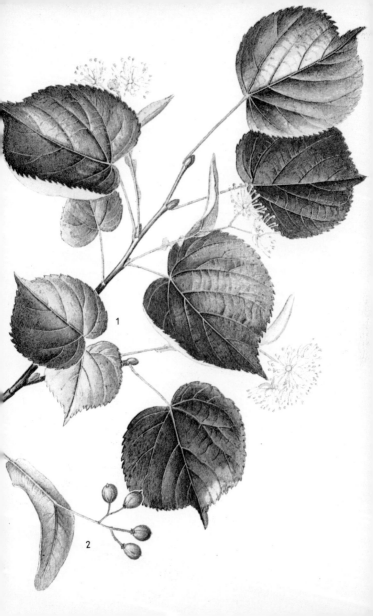

1

2

Tropaeolum majus L.

Tropaeolaceae

Nasturtium

This perennial herb, which under cultivation is an annual, flowers from May to September. It is native to South America (Peru and Bolivia) and is established on the Juan Fernandez Islands off Chile. Countless cultivars, differing in the colour of the crown, are cultivated as ornamentals in gardens and parks, and occasionally the plant grows wild in Madeira, Europe, China and Brazil. In 1684 it was introduced into central Europe by the Dutchman Bewerning.

The parts used for pharmaceutical purposes are the seeds *(Semen tropaeoli)*. The fruit is collected as it becomes ripe during August and September, whereupon it is dried in a well-ventilated spot and divested of the seed. The drug smells like potatoes, is tasteless at first but later causes a sharp burning sensation on the tongue. It contains a glycoside — which on fermentation is converted into an essential oil — and a highly efficient but unstable antibiotic. These active principles have a pronounced and broad antibacterial and antimycotic effect.

The seeds are used internally in crushed form, generally coated with sugar, in the treatment of inflammation of the urinary passages caused by infection, in bronchitis and for influenza. The seeds are a component of several specifics. Besides the drug, the flowers, leaves and also the juice of fresh plants are used as a popular home remedy. *Tropaeolum* is cultivated for pharmaceutical purposes. Collection of the fruits is difficult, however, mainly because of the long flowering period and the irregular ripening of the seed, which results in a high percentage of loss in the harvested crop.

1. *Flowering plant*
2. *Fruit*

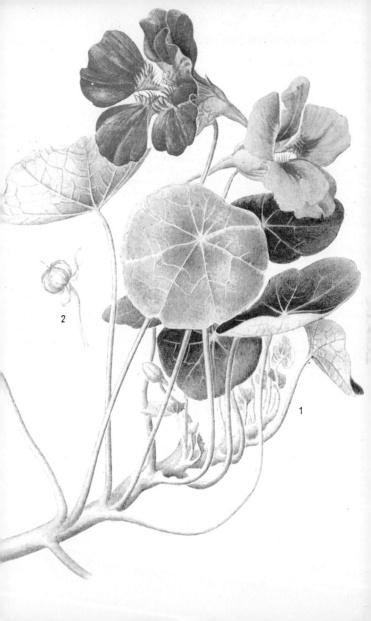

Tussilago farfara L.

Coltsfoot

Coltsfoot is a perennial herb flowering from March to May. It is native to Europe, North Africa, northern and western Asia, and has been introduced into America. It grows in abundance on loamy, moist soils, in hedgerows and in barren places.

The parts collected for the drug market are the inflorescence *(Flos farfarae)* and the leaves *(Folium farfarae)*. The flowers are gathered from March to April before they have passed their prime. The leaves are gathered whole from May to July. Care should be taken that they are not damaged or attacked by disease or pests. The flowers, divested of the stalk, are dried at temperatures not exceeding 40° C as are the leaves; the latter may also be dried in the sun. The drugs are odourless and have a mucilaginous, slightly bitter taste. They contain a large quantity of mucilage, a minute amount of tannins and probably also saponins, and exert an expectorant as well as disinfectant and anti-inflammatory action.

The drugs are used internally as an infusion or in herbal teas in treatment of the common cold and cough, and externally in the form of compresses in the treatment of varicose veins, varicose ulcers and certain types of exuding rashes.

The drugs are gathered only in the wild. When collecting the leaves great care must be taken not to gather those of certain species of *Petasites* MILL. which show a marked resemblance.

1. *Inflorescences*
2. *Young leaves*

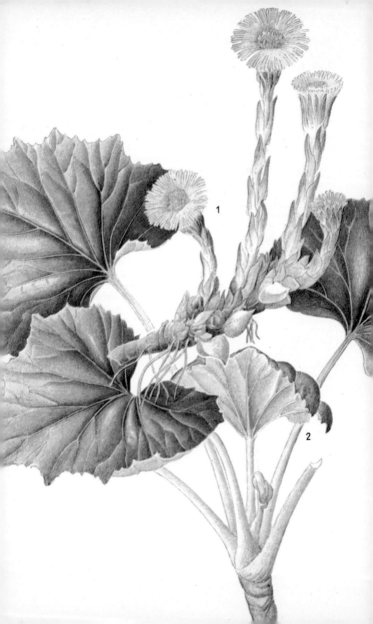

Vaccinium myrtillus L.

Ericaceae

Blueberry

A shrub, flowering from April to July, the Blueberry grows fairly abundantly, often in masses, in woods and marshes from hilly to alpine elevations — sometimes even above the line of continuous dwarf pine growths. It occurs in the arctic and temperate regions of the Northern Hemisphere, with the possible exception of northern Asia. In the south its distribution is confined mostly to hills. It is absent from Greece and the Atlas Mountains of Morocco.

The parts used for extraction of the active principles are the dried fruits *(Fructus myrtilli)* and leaves *(Folium myrtilli)*. The fruits are gathered when ripe and dried in the shade or in the sun. When artificial heat is used the temperature must not exceed 45° C. The berries must be dried thoroughly for otherwise they become mouldy. The dry fruits are odourless and cause an astringent sensation on the tongue. The leaves, collected between June and September, are stripped from the stalks and dried in the same manner as the fruits. The berries contain as much as 10 per cent of tannins and a large amount of sugars, pectins, organic acids and pigments. They exert an astringent and costive action in the intestines. The leaves also contain tannins and other little known substances reducing the sugar level in the blood. They have a mild disinfectant effect in infections of the kidney and bladder. In some cases they reduce the blood sugar level in diabetes.

The fruits are popularly used in the form of a decoction for diarrhoea, and also as a gargle for stomatitis. The decoction from the leaves and seedcoats of the berries is an efficient subsidiary medicine in the treatment of diabetes. The berries, however, are used far more widely as a food.

The drug is collected only in the wild. The berries were listed as a medicinal drug by Abbess Hildegarde of Germany as early as the twelfth century.

1. *Fruit-bearing branch*
2. *Branch with flowers*

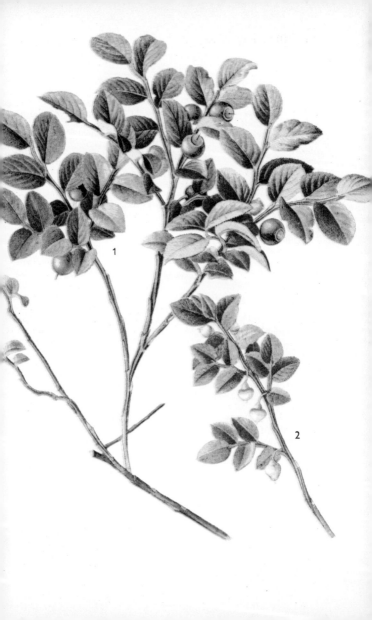

Valeriana officinalis L.

Valerianaceae

Valerian

This perennial herb, flowering from May to September, grows sparsely to fairly abundantly on damp meadows and shrub-covered slopes, in coastal thickets, pastureland and ditches, and alongside waterways from lowland to subalpine elevations. It is distributed throughout the temperate regions of Eurasia and has been introduced into North America. Valerian has been known for its medicinal properties since 924 AD; it was first mentioned by Isaac Judaes.

The parts collected for drug production are the rhizomes and roots (*Radix valerianae*) of cultivated plants, generally second-year though sometimes also first-year growths. These are always gathered in the autumn, then thoroughly washed and dried by artificial heat at temperatures up to 45° C. The drug acquires an aromatic odour only after drying. The flavour is sweet and spicy and slightly bitter at the same time. It contains about 1 per cent of an essential oil rich in various constituents, which in isolation have practically no therapeutic effect but are very efficient as a combined group. The drug has a sedative effect on neurogenic irritability, a beneficial action on heart disorders of nervous origin and alleviates spasms.

It is used internally in macerated form, as a tincture and in precisely dosed pharmaceutical preparations and specifics as a general sedative in insomnia caused by nervous exhaustion, increased heart rate and agitation.

Valerian is cultivated mainly in Germany, the Netherlands, Belgium and countries of eastern Europe, chiefly the USSR.

1. *Part of a flowering stem*
2. *Detail of flower*
3. *Rhizome and roots*

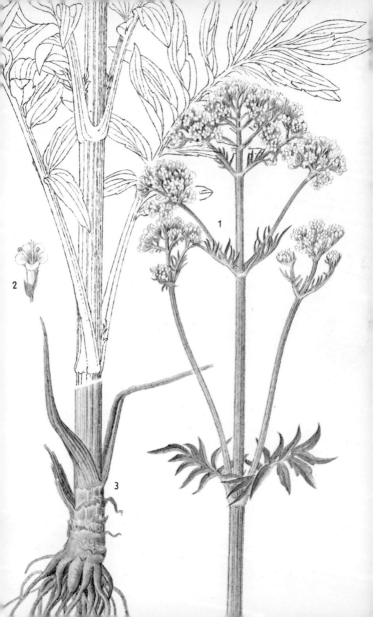

† *Veratrum album* L.

Liliaceae

European White Hellebore

This is a perennial herb which flowers from June to August and has a thin to fairly abundant distribution in meadows and forest clearings, on hillsides and among rough grass from foothill to alpine elevations, rarely at lower altitudes. It is distributed throughout the temperate regions of Eurasia. Green Hellebore *(Veratrum viride* AIT.*)* is found in the temperate regions of North America.

The parts collected for medicinal purposes are the rhizomes *(Radix veratri)* which are gathered in autumn. After being washed and cut into pieces they are dried in a shaded, well-ventilated spot or with artificial heat at a temperature of 45° C. The drug is odourless, has a sharp, bitter taste and provokes fits of sneezing. It must be remembered that the plant is extremely toxic and great care must be taken in its collection. The drug contains numerous alkaloids, closely related to certain glycosidic alkaloids of *Solanum nigrum* L. and to some extent structurally related to the cardiac glycosides. The alkaloids act as a respiratory depressant, cause increased salivation, thirst and retching.

The drug is little used in human medicine; the pure alkaloids are very occasionally used in the treatment of certain diseases and hypertension. Today the drug serves mainly for the isolation of pure alkaloids which are used in a limited number of pharmaceutical specifics. It is of far greater importance in veterinary medicine where it is employed internally in digestive disorders of livestock and externally against certain parasites.

1. *Rhizome*
2. *Flowering top part*

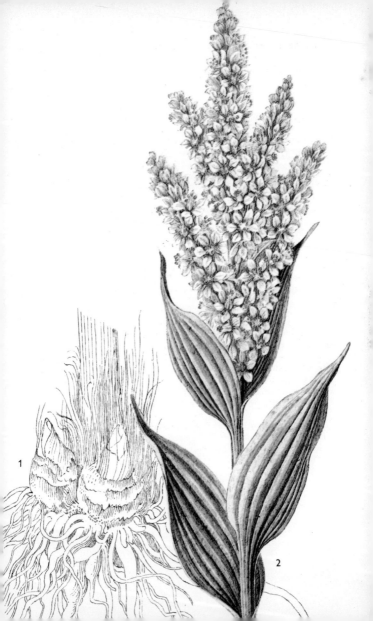

Verbascum thapsiforme SCHRAD.   Scrophulariaceae

Mullein

This is a biennial herb flowering from July to September and fairly abundant on sunny hillsides and scree, on stony riverbanks and pastures from lowland to foothill elevations in warmer climates. It is distributed throughout Europe (except in the northernmost areas, the south-western parts of the Iberian Peninsula and the Alps) and in the Caucasus.

The parts collected for medicinal purposes are the golden-yellow flower petals and stamens *(Flos verbasci)* which are gathered as they open, always in dry weather. Care must be taken not to crush the petals as this makes them turn brown and decreases the value of the crude drug. They should be dried carefully in thin layers in the shade; they may require a further period of drying by artificial heat at a temperature not exceeding 40° C, and can then be stored in air-tight containers, best of all in sealed tins, as they easily absorb moisture, turn brown and lose their efficacy. The drug has an agreeable honey-like smell and taste. It contains saponins, which have not yet been fully investigated, mucilage, flavonoids, traces of an essential oil and sugars. These substances have a beneficial effect on the symptoms of diseases associated with chilling for they exert an expectorant action and diminish the cough reflex. The probable presence of antibiotic substances gives the drug its anti-inflammatory properties.

The drug is used internally in the form of an infusion in cough and mucous congestion. It is generally a component of herbal teas used in the treatment of chest colds, and also in other tea mixtures to which its colour imparts a more attractive appearance.

It is collected wild but also cultivated as a field crop. The burden of collecting and preparing the drug makes the output rather small and as it is much in demand it is fairly expensive. The flowers of another European species *Verbascum phlomoides* L., which is widespread in similar habitats, are also collected.

1. *Top part of stem with inflorescence*
2. *Leaves*
    Both 1. and 2. are from a plant in its second year.

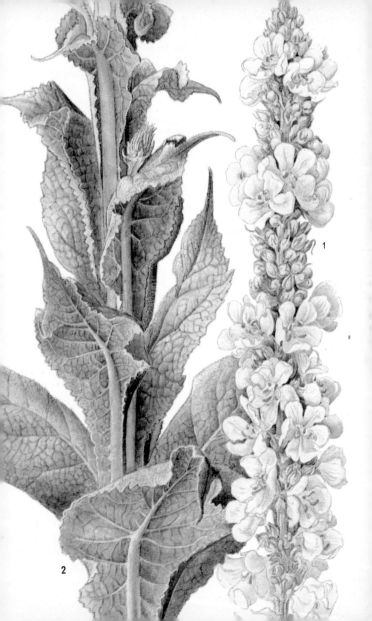

Viola odorata L.

Sweet Violet

This is a perennial herb, flowering from March to May, which grows fairly freely in hedgebanks, scrub and shady spots in damp woods, usually on calcareous soils from lowland to foothill elevations. It is often cultivated as an ornamental and found growing wild in gardens and parks. *Viola odorata* is in all probability indigenous only to the Mediterranean countries and in the area extending from western Europe to southern England. It has long since become established throughout most of Europe and has also been introduced into eastern Asia and North America. Closely related species are found in southern and eastern Asia.

The rhizomes *(Radix violae odoratae)* are collected for medicinal purposes from September to October. They are first washed and then dried in a well-ventilated and shady spot or with artificial heat at temperatures not exceeding 45° C. The drug is odourless and causes a sharp burning sensation on the tongue. It contains saponins and the glycoside of salicylic acid. It exerts an expectorant action, and also has a diuretic effect.

It is used internally in the form of an infusion or as a component of herbal tea mixtures used to relieve bronchitis and coughing. In pediatrics it is often employed in cough syrups. The drug's diuretic properties are employed in rheumatic diseases. Externally, it is used in gargles.

The drug is collected only in the wild. On the Riviera it is cultivated for use in perfumery. It has been known since ancient times; both Hippocrates and Pliny make reference to its virtues.

Flowering plant

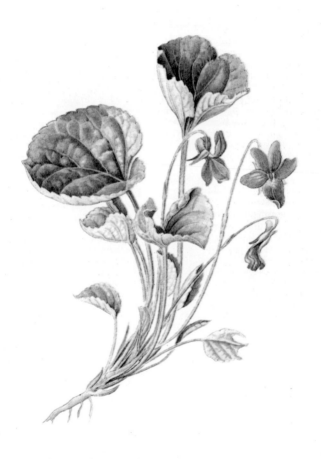

Viola tricolor L.

Violaceae

Heartsease, Wild Pansy

This is an annual to perennial herb which flowers from May to October and grows freely in fields, meadows, hedgerows and waste land from lowland to foothill elevations. It is distributed in the temperate regions of Eurasia as far east as the Altai and south-west India, south to the Mediterranean and to Iceland in the north.

The flower heads *(Herba violae tricoloris)* are collected for the drug market in May to September, minus the lower parts of the stalks. They are dried in thin layers in the shade or with artificial heat at temperatures not exceeding 45° C. When drying care should be taken that the flowers do not absorb any moisture during the process for this causes a change in colour and probably also a loss in the efficiency of the active principles. The drug is odourless and has a sweetish, mucilaginous taste. It contains saponins, flavones and salicylic acid compounds. It has an expectorant and diuretic effect, and stimulates metabolism and secretion of the sweat glands.

It is used internally in the form of an infusion or as a component of herbal teas for the relief of catarrh of the respiratory passages accompanied by fever, for inflammation of the urinary bladder and prostate gland, and to stimulate the metabolism in rheumatism and gout. Externally it is employed as a gargle and also in compresses, or as a bath preparation in the treatment of certain skin rashes. If taken over a long period, however, patients sensitive to salicylic preparations may show allergic reactions in the form of a rash.

The drug is collected only in the wild. In mediaeval times, however, it was sometimes cultivated as well.

Flowering plant

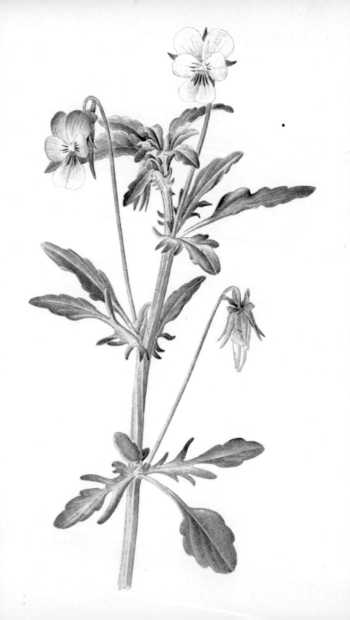

† *Viscum album* L.

Loranthaceae

Mistletoe

This is a somewhat woody evergreen, parasitic on the branches of trees, which flowers from March to April. It is found on a great variety of deciduous trees from lowland to foothill elevations, sometimes up to alpine elevations, but is particularly common on apple trees; it grows much more rarely on evergreens and conifers. It is distributed in central and southern England, southern Scandinavia, central Europe, the Mediterranean countries, Iran, the Himalayas, Tibet, the northern parts of south-east Asia, China and Japan. In Eurasia it has a discontinuous distribution and in Algeria it occurs in isolated localities.

The branches and leaves *(Stipes et Folium visci)*, are gathered for medicinal purposes in the winter months. They are dried at temperatures up to 45° C. The drug has a faint but distinctive odour and bitter taste. Its chief constituent is a toxin but it also contains traces of alkaloids in addition to other active principles. Specific effects are the lowering of blood pressure and a cardiac action; the drug is also known to have mild diuretic properties. Experiments on mice have shown that it inhibits malignant growths, but this has not yet been proved in humans.

The drug is used internally as a maceration, as an extract or as a component of pharmaceutical specifics used in the treatment of hypertension, arteriosclerosis and diseases of nervous origin. Some physicians consider Mistletoe preparations as possible medicaments in the treatment of cancer patients where surgery is no longer a possibility.

Mistletoe is only collected in the wild. Sometimes *Loranthus europaeus* L., which resembles Mistletoe, is collected by mistake. Classifying the various forms of Mistletoe according to the host on which they live is possible but does not appear to have any medical significance.

1. *Branch with flowers*
2. *Branch with fruits*
3. *Female flowers*
4. *Male flowers*

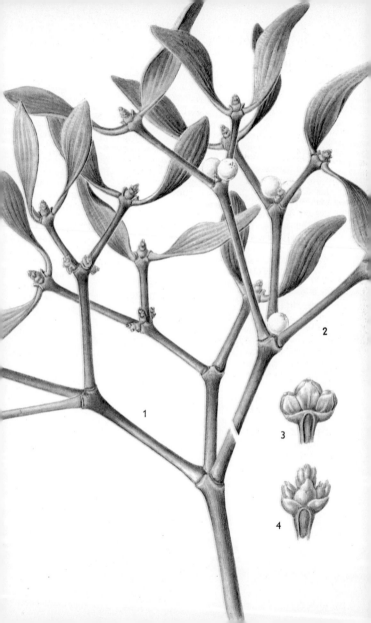

1

2

3

4

GLOSSARY

Active principle — the chemical component responsible for the physiological effects of a drug plant

Acute — intense and of brief duration

Adventitious root — a root arising not as part of the organised rooting system but as and where required, often from aerial portions of a plant

Alcoholic extract — an alcoholic solution of active principles obtained by steeping the drug in alcohol

Alkaloid — a nitrogen-containing, organic, basic compound occurring in plants. The alkaloids include such substances as atropine, nicotine and quinine

Allergy — an exaggerated reaction or sensitivity of an organism to a certain substance (which may be a medical remedy)

Amino acid — a fatty acid containing a substituted amino group. Amino acids are important as the elements from which proteins are built

Anaesthesia — the loss of sensation

Analgesic — pain-relieving; a remedy which relieves pain

Annual — living for a single season; an annual plant

Anodyne — a medicine which relieves distressful symptoms

Anthelmintic — removing worms; a remedy which is used for combatting worms

Antibiotic — inhibiting the growth of germs; a substance which inhibits the growth of germs. Penicillin, the first antibiotic to be used in medicine, was discovered by Sir Alexander Fleming

Anticoagulant — a substance which prevents blood from clotting

Antimycotic — a substance which checks fungal growth

Antispasmodic — a remedy which prevents muscular spasm

Aromatic — fragrant, stimulating the senses of taste and smell

Arteriosclerosis — a hardening of the walls of the arteries

Astringent — causing local contraction of skin and constriction of blood vessels and checking secretion; a substance with such an action

Auxilliary medicine — a medicine which increases the effect of another medicine when taken with it

Biennial — living for two seasons; a plant with a life-cycle of two seasons. During the first season's growth food is produced and stored; the plant flowers and bears fruit in the second season

Bitter principle — the chemical component of a plant responsible for its bitter taste

Bulb — a modified bud with persistent fleshy leaf bases, usually underground. Certain perennial plants survive the winter as bulbs. The fleshy leaf bases act as storage organs

Capsule — a dry, usually many-seeded fruit which splits to shed its contents

Carbohydrate — a chemical compound made up of the elements carbon, hydrogen and oxygen. Simple sugars, such as glucose and fructose, and polysaccharides, such as starch and pectin, are examples of carbohydrates

Carcinogen — a substance which tends to produce cancer

Carminative — relieving flatulence; a carminative medicine

226

Catabolism — the process or processes leading to the chemical breakdown of substances within the body

Catarrh — the inflammation of a mucous membrane, such as that lining the nasal cavity or stomach, leading to excessive secretion of mucus

Cathartic — evacuating the bowels, purgative

Chronic — of long duration (as opposed to acute)

Colic — a paroxysm of acute abdominal pain

Corm — a swollen, underground rootstock, similar in function to a bulb

Costive — producing constipation

Coumarin — a fragrant, aromatic compound common in plant tissues. Coumarin is largely responsible for the scent of new-mown hay. Although coumarin itself has little pharmacological activity, its derivatives are often anticoagulants

Cultivar — a plant variety that has been produced under cultivation

Cytostatic — preventing cell division, often with reference to malignant or tumorous cells

Decoction — an extract prepared by boiling the crude drug in water, or by pouring boiling water over it and allowing it to stand

Depressant — lowering the level or slowing the rate of activity; a sedative

Dermatitis — an inflammation of the skin

Dermatosis — a disease of the skin

Digestion — an extract prepared by steeping the crude drug in warm water (35—40 °C.)

227

Diuretic — promoting and increasing the flow of urine

Dyspepsia — the impaired digestion of food

Enzyme — a complex protein that brings about or accelerates chemical reactions

Essential oil — a volatile oil obtained from a plant, possessing the smell and other characteristic properties of the plant

Expectorant — promoting the discharge of matter from the throat or lungs by coughing; a drug with such an effect

Flatulence — the presence of gas in the gut

Flavone — an organic, yellow pigment occurring in many animal and plant tissues

Fruit — the ripened ovary of a plant containing the seed or seeds

Furocoumarin — a glycoside compounded of coumarin and furanose

Glycoside — a substance in which a simple sugar is combined with another organic compound

Haemolysis — the breakdown of red blood cells. The cell walls rupture releasing the cell contents

Haemorrhage — the loss of blood from an internal or external wound or lesion

Haemorrhoid — a mass of dilated veins under the skin of the anus

Haemostatic — arresting loss of blood; a substance which staunches bleeding

228

Hepatitis — an inflammation of the liver

Herb — a flowering plant whose parts above ground do not persist from one season to the next; a plant used for medicinal or culinary purposes

Hormone — a substance produced by a ductless gland and distributed through the body by the circulating blood to the organs which it affects

Hydrolysis — the breakdown of a chemical substance into simpler components by the addition of water

Hygroscopic — absorbing moisture from the air

Hypertension — a state of abnormally high blood pressure

Hypotension — a state of abnormally low blood pressure

Infarction — a small area of body tissue which has died because the blood vessel supplying it has become blocked

Inflorescence — a stem axis bearing flowers

Infusion — an extract obtained by steeping the drug in water

Invert sugar — the mixture of sugars (glucose and fructose) which results from the hydrolysis of cane sugar (sucrose)

Lactation — the formation and secretion of milk

Lanatoside — a glycoside which occurs particularly in *Digitalis lanata*

Lichen — a primitive plant consisting of algal and fungal cells in close association

Liniment — a liquid pharmaceutical preparation for external use, usually oily, and applied by rubbing

Maceration — the extraction of constituents from a drug by steeping it in water at room temperature for several hours

Metabolism — the chemical processes taking place within living organisms which provide energy, incorporate new material and break down unwanted substances

Mucilage — a gel-like polysaccharide present in certain plant tissues

Narcotic — having a numbing or sleep-inducing effect; a narcotic drug (such as cocaine, morphine)

Neuritis — the inflammation of a nerve or nerves

Non-specific — having a general effect, not restricted to a single organ, function, etc.

Oedema — the swelling up of a part of the body due to accumulation of excess tissue fluid

Oestrogen — a hormone (actually more than one substance) produced by the ovary and influencing the female reproductive organs

Organic acid — an acid occurring in the tissues of living organisms

Paediatrics — the study and treatment of the diseases of children

Pectin — a mixture of complex carbohydrates found in the cell walls of plants

Perennial — having a life-cycle lasting more than two seasons; a perennial plant

Peristalsis — the rhythmic, wave-like contraction of smooth muscle lining tubular structures like the gut and seminal vesicles. In the gut, peristalsis serves to agitate food, thus aiding its digestion, and to move food along the gut.

Pharmaceutics — the science of preparing and dispensing drugs and medicines

Pharmacognosy — the study of the biological sources, chemistry and pharmacology of plant-derived drugs

Pharmacology — the study of the effects of chemical substance on animal tissues

Phytochemistry — the study of the chemistry and biochemistry of plants

Polysaccharide — a complex carbohydrate consisting of a number of simple sugars chemically linked together. Polysaccharides can be broken down into their component sugars by hydrolysis

Proteolysis — the breakdown of proteins by hydrolysis into their component amino acids

Resin — a complex substance found in plants, usually as an exudate, which is insoluble and aromatic, and chemically related to the terpenes

Rhizome — an elongated underground stem. A rhizome may be an organ of storage and an overwintering structure.

Rootstock — the persistent basal part of the stem in some perennial herbs from which new roots and shoots arise at each growing season

Saponin — a glycoside found in plant tissues which has the property of lowering the surface tension of water and hence causing foaming. Saponins cause haemolysis and are also highly poisonous to fish

Sclerosis — the pathological hardening of body tissue

Sedative — having a soothing or sleep-producing action; a sedative drug

Seed — a ripened ovule, containing an embryonic plant

Shrub — a woody plant which branches near to the ground

Smooth muscle — a type of muscle tissue, distinguishable from striped (voluntary) muscle and cardiac muscle by its microscopic structure, which is outside direct voluntary control. Smooth muscle is capable of sustained contraction or prolonged rhythmic activity and occurs in such organs as the bladder, gut and uterus.

Spasm — an intense, uncontrolled muscular contraction

Specific — having a special effect in the treatment of a particular disease; a specific medicine

Spore — a walled structure, containing one or more cells each of which is capable of producing a phase of the life-cycle

Stigma — the part of a plant's female reproductive organs which is concerned with the reception of pollen

Stimulant — raising the level of or accelerating activity; a stimulant drug

Stomachic — beneficial to the stomach or stimulating the digestion; a stomachic medicine

Stomatitis — an inflammation of the mouth

Sugar — a carbohydrate of low molecular weight, soluble in water and usually with a sweet taste

Synergism — the combined action of two drugs such that their individual effects are enhanced

Systemic — affecting the body as a whole

Tannin — a plant-derived substance with astringent properties. Tannins occur particularly in Oak bark and are used in processing leather

Terpene — a compound built up around one or more similar chemical units (isoprene). Terpenes range from camphor to rubber (a polyterpene) and include the resins.

Thallus — the body of a primitive plant, undifferentiated into root and shoot and lacking tissue specialized for transporting nutrients

Tincture — a solution of active principles prepared by extraction in alcohol

Tonic — invigorating or strengthening; a tonic medicine

Toxic — poisonous

Toxin — a poison, especially a substance of organic origin

Trace element — a chemical element — especially iodine, copper, cobalt, manganese, zinc and molybdenum — whose presence, albeit in minute amounts, is essential to living organisms

Tuber — the swollen tip of an underground stem

Urology — the study and treatment of diseases of the urino-genital tract

Vasodilator — relaxing or expanding blood vessels; a vasodilator drug

Vitamin — a complex substance of organic origin which in small quantities is necessary for the maintenance of animal life

Volatile oil — an essential oil distilled from plant tissue characterized by the readiness with which it evaporates

Xerophyte — a plant which grows in dry conditions

BIBLIOGRAPHY

British Herbal Medical Association, *British Herbal Pharmacopoeia*, London, 1971.

Chopra, R.N., Ed., *Indigenous Drugs of India* (U.N. Dhur & Sons), Calcutta, 1968.

Claus, E.P. and Tyler, V. E., *Pharmacognosy* (H. Kimpton), London, 1965.

Crow, W.B., *The Occult Properties of Herbs* (Aquarian Press), London, 1969.

Emboden, W., *Narcotic Plants* (Studio Vista), London, 1971.

Hemphill, R., *Penguin Book of Herbs and Spices* (Penguin Books), London, 1966.

Krieg, M.B., *Green Medicine* (R. McNally & Co.), New York, 1964.

Meyer, J.E., *The Herbalist*, Revized Edition (Sterling Publishing Co.), New York, 1968.

Ministry of Agriculture, Fisheries and Food, *British Poisonous Plants*, Bull. No 161 (H.M.S.O.), London, 1968.

Schofield, M., *The Strange Case of Pot* (Penguin Books), London, 1971.

Taylor, N.E., *Plant Drugs that Changed the World* (Allen & Unwin), London, 1966.

Todd, R.G., Ed. *Extra Pharmacopoeia*, 25th Edition (Pharmaceutical Press), London, 1967.

Trease, G.E., and Evans, W.C., *Pharmacognosy*, 10th Edition (Bailliere Tindall), London, 1971.

Watt, J.M., and Breyen-Bradwijk, M.G., *The Medicinal and Poisonous Plants of Southern and Eastern Africa* (E. and S. Livingston), London, 1962.

Wren, R. C. and Wren, R.W., *Potter's New Cyclopaedia of Botanical Drugs and Preparations* (Potter & Clark), London, 1968.

INDEX OF COMMON NAMES

INDEX OF LATIN NAMES